the anti-anxiety food solution

How the Foods You Eat Can Help You Calm Your Anxious Mind, Improve Your Mood & End Cravings

TRUDY SCOTT, CN

New Harbinger Publications, Inc.

Publisher's Note

Every effort is made to ensure that the information contained in this book is complete and accurate. Neither the publisher nor the author is engaged in rendering professional advice to the reader. The information and suggestions provided in this book are not intended as a substitute for advice from your physician. All matters regarding health require medical supervision. Neither the author nor the publisher shall be liable for any injury or damage allegedly arising from any information or suggestions in this book. Recommendations, including for supplements, are intended only as guidelines; needs of individuals will vary. The opinions expressed in this book represent the personal views of the author and not the publisher. The author is a practitioner of nutrition and not a licensed physician, and does not diagnose or prescribe.

"The Four-Part Mood-Type Questionnaire" & "Caution Box", adapted from THE MOOD CURE by Julia Ross, copyright © 2002 by Julia Ross. Used by permission of Viking Penguin, a division of Penguin Group (USA) Inc.

Distributed in Canada by Raincoast Books

New Harbinger Publications, Inc.
5674 Shattuck Avenue
Oakland, CA 94609
www.newharbinger.com

Cover design by Amy Shoup
Acquired by Jess O'Brien
Edited by Jasmine Star

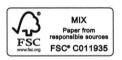

MIX
Paper from responsible sources
FSC® C011935
www.fsc.org

Library of Congress Cataloging-in-Publication Data

Scott, Trudy, 1960-
The antianxiety food solution : how the foods you eat can help you calm your anxious mind, improve your mood, and end cravings / Trudy Scott.
    p. cm.
Includes bibliographical references.
ISBN 978-1-57224-925-7 (pbk.) -- ISBN 978-1-57224-926-4 (PDF ebook)
1. Anxiety disorders--Diet therapy. 2. Nutrition--Psychological aspects. I. Title.
RC531.S36 2011
616.85'220654--dc22

                                        2011007069

Printed in the United States of America

21   20   19

20   19   18   17   16

"Trudy Scott's book, *The Antianxiety Food Solution*, fills an important gap in the popular literature on anxiety. It provides clear, helpful guidelines for utilizing nutrition to overcome anxiety."

—Edmund Bourne, PhD, author of *The Anxiety and Phobia Workbook*

"A great book with plenty of practical advice backed by science."

—Daniel G. Amen, MD, author of *Change Your Brain, Change Your Life*

"Every one of the millions now suffering from anxiety has a new friend in Trudy Scott, whose book offers them a nutritional lifeline. Replete with specific and practical suggestions, this book is backed up by research and clinical expertise."

—Julia Ross, MA, MFT, author of *The Mood Cure* and *The Diet Cure*

"This book is a must-read if you have anxiety and want to treat the underlying causes and heal, rather than having to rely on medications. Adjust your brain chemistry with the right nutrients and you can reclaim your brain and your life!"

—Hyla Cass, MD, author of *8 Weeks to Vibrant Health*

"This book is a real tour-de-force in complementary mental health literature and should be on the shelves of every anxiety sufferer. It's a user-friendly and balanced book about foods and nutrients that can reduce anxiety, and it is also refreshingly original."

—Jonathan Prousky, MSc, ND, professor of clinical nutrition at the Canadian College of Naturopathic Medicine and author of *Anxiety: Orthomolecular Diagnosis and Treatment*

"As a nutrition and fitness expert and the mother of a child with an emotional disorder, I find this book invaluable. It is one I will use myself and recommend to both clients and colleagues."

—JJ Virgin, CNS, CHFS, nutrition and fitness expert, author of *Six Weeks to Sleeveless and Sexy*, and cohost of TLC's *Freaky Eaters*

"A leader in the field of food and mental health, Trudy Scott supplements the core themes of food and gut health with chapters on amino acids, pyroluria, and lifestyle changes. Trudy aptly emphasizes that readers should try to find the root cause of their health problems."

—Lawrence E. Cormier, MD, holistic psychiatrist in Denver, CO

"This book may be the key you've been looking for. It does an excellent job of explaining the science behind anxiety and then bringing it to a practical level, providing a nutritional and integrative approach to anxiety."

—Elizabeth Lipski, PhD, CCN, director of doctoral studies at Hawthorn University in Whitethorn, CA, and author of *Digestive Wellness*

"Trudy Scott's work communicates something I tell my patients every day: there is a powerful connection between what we eat and how we feel."

—Mike Dow, PsyD, cohost of TLC's *Freaky Eaters*

"I recommend this book not only to those who suffer from anxiety, but to their health care providers as well."

> —Karla Maree, certified nutrition consultant, neuronutrient therapist, and director of nutritional therapy at Recovery Systems Clinic

"A comprehensive book providing the nation with much-needed formulas for overcoming anxiety and restoring stable emotions!"

> —Joan Mathews-Larson, PhD, LADC, founder of the Health Recovery Center in Minneapolis, MN, and author of *Depression-Free, Naturally*

"This book offers a wealth of useful information for those who would like to try dietary and other lifestyle changes in order to improve their mental health. It is also a valuable resource for clinicians interested in broadening their approach to the treatment of anxiety."

> —Felice N. Jacka, PhD, research fellow at the University of Melbourne in Australia

"I am impressed by how thorough this book is. I also love the combination of the text and the tables, which makes it easy to follow."

> —Bonnie Fisk-Hayden, MS, nutritional consultant and board member of National Association of Nutrition Professionals

"An easy-to-read book that should help many people with anxiety."

> —Michael B. Schachter, MD, CNS, board-certified psychiatrist

"Full of practical tips for restoring balance to your body and mind. I highly recommend it."

> —Mark Atkinson, MD, author of *The Mind-Body Bible*

"*The Antianxiety Food Solution* is one of the most comprehensive guides to nutritional healing for anxiety."

> —Elizabeth Large, ND

"I am really looking forward to sharing this book and wealth of information with friends and patients."

> —Wendy Young, occupational therapist in Durban, South Africa

"This book should be on the bookshelves of everyone who wants to take back control of their health. I'm so glad to have this book as a resource!"

> —Jessica Sitomer, professional speaker and author

"Trudy Scott is an expert on the relationship between food and mood, an often neglected area. This book provides clearly presented practical information, which I believe to be important adjunctive help in the treatment anxiety, depression, and serious mental illness."

> —Katherine Falk, MD, psychiatrist in New York, NY

For everyone suffering from anxiety and looking for answers. And for all the nutritionists, holistic health professionals, and researchers who are making a difference in the field of nutrition and mental health.

Acknowledgments

Thanks to the following peer reviewers: Bonnie Fisk-Hayden, MS; Elizabeth Lipski, PhD, CCN; Karla Maree, CNC; James Lake, MD; Joan Mathews-Larson, PhD, Mikell Susanne Parsons, DC; Julia Ross, MA; and Michael Schachter, MD, CNS.

Thanks to my wonderful copyeditor, Jasmine Star.

Thanks to everyone behind the scenes who contributed to this end result.

Thanks to my mom, who helped so much with the initial typing—and thanks for feeding us kids real whole food!

Last but not least, thanks to my wonderful husband, Brad, for your love and support, for making me laugh every single day, and for all the fun we have!

Contents

Foreword

Many people who are diagnosed with a psychiatric disorder rely on nonpharmacologic therapies alone or in combination with conventional drug treatment. In the United States, Canada, and Europe, treatments other than prescription medications and psychotherapy are regarded as complementary and alternative medicine (CAM). In addition to herbs and vitamins, dietary changes are generally regarded as a kind of CAM therapy. It is estimated that approximately 10 percent of U.S. adults who visit a CAM practitioner have a psychiatric diagnosis, and half of those are seeking care primarily for their mental health problem (Druss and Rosenheck 2000). Over half of individuals diagnosed with an anxiety or mood disorder use CAM therapies, including natural supplements and dietary changes (Kessler et al. 2001).

Widespread and increasing use of nonpharmacologic therapies is occurring in the context of growing concern about the adequacy of conventional drug treatments for mental health problems. After decades of studies and billions of dollars of pharmaceutical industry funding, the best research findings suggest that conventional prescription medications are only marginally superior—if not equivalent—to placebos for the treatment of psychiatric disorders. Given the unresolved safety concerns associated with psychotropic drugs, there are compelling reasons to explore promising nonpharmacologic approaches, including simple changes in lifestyle and nutrition. In parallel with these concerns, research findings are supporting the use of select CAM therapies as safe and effective treatments of common psychiatric disorders, including anxiety disorders. Together, all of these factors have led to increasing openness to nonpharmacologic treatments among health care providers, researchers, and patients.

Physicians often advise their patients about reasonable dietary changes for the prevention and treatment of medical illnesses such as heart disease and diabetes; however, mental health professionals often overlook the importance of nutrition for both maintaining good mental health and treating specific mental health problems. Trudy Scott has wisely chosen to focus on a major mental health problem that has not been adequately addressed by contemporary biomedical psychiatry, as evidenced by the high rate of anxiety disorders in the general population, the limited effectiveness of conventional pharmacologic treatments for these disorders, and the significant safety issues associated with commonly used antianxiety drugs.

Anxiety in particular is a common problem in the general population. Established conventional treatments for anxiety include cognitive-behavioral therapy and psychopharmacology. Regarding the latter, medications alone do not adequately address the root causes of anxiety. And as mentioned, there are concerns in regard to both safety and effectiveness. One analysis that reviewed a number of high-quality studies showed that the effectiveness of pharmacologic and psychotherapeutic treatments varies widely depending on the severity and type of anxiety (Westen and Morrison 2001). Although sedative-hypnotic drugs and serotonin reuptake inhibitors can help in the short-term treatment of panic attacks and generalized anxiety, most patients remain symptomatic over the long term (Westen and Morrison 2001). Further, patients who chronically use potent sedative-hypnotic drugs to control severe anxiety symptoms, including social anxiety and panic attacks, are at significant risk of becoming dependent on these drugs and experiencing withdrawal when they discontinue the medication. In addition, most psychotropic drugs cause significant weight gain and frequently lead to obesity (Schwartz et al. 2004).

Trudy Scott's book marks an important contribution to the public dialogue on the appropriate role of nutrition in mental health care in general and anxiety disorders in particular. When approaching any medical or psychiatric disorder, there is no intervention more fundamental than sound advice on nutrition. In this book,

Trudy Scott establishes a compelling case for the benefits of rational nutritional choices in the prevention and treatment of anxiety disorders. I strongly endorse this unique resource and recommend it without reservation to both conventionally trained and alternative medical practitioners, as well as everyone who has tried conventional pharmacologic treatment or psychotherapy and continues to struggle with anxiety.

—James Lake, MD
President of the International Network of Integrative Mental Health
Author of *Textbook of Integrative Mental Health Care*

Introduction

You are a smart, capable person—successful and dynamic, with a can-do attitude. You achieve great things and have an amazing family and a wonderful life. Suddenly you are brought to your knees. Many a morning you wake terrified, with a pounding heart, anxious and fearful of who knows what—there is no reason! Sometimes, out of the blue, your throat constricts and you feel helpless, waiting for that awful feeling to subside. Other times you barely manage to get through your day, smiling and chatting bravely, with absurd feelings of pending doom and gloom—for absolutely no reason. These panic attacks are scary. You feel frozen in time, you can hardly breathe, and your racing heart feels as if it will explode. You even begin to feel anxious about when the next panic attack will strike. You may worry excessively, feel overwhelmed, and have stiff, tense muscles. Social events are the worst. When you run out of excuses, you force yourself to participate, but it's painful, and you wonder if others will see through your fragile facade. You wonder, *What's going on? Am I crazy? Am I losing it? What should I do? Should I tell someone? Where do I turn?*

If there's no obvious reason for your anxiety, chances are lifestyle and biochemistry play a role. The guidelines you'll discover in this book will help you repair your biochemistry, balance your neurotransmitters, and nourish your body so you can eliminate your anxiety and panic attacks, and feel calm, relaxed, and worry free.

My Story

There's a reason why I'm so passionate about working with people who have anxiety and why I'm writing this book. I've had my own personal journey with anxiety, starting in my midthirties. My anxiety was just like the previous description: feelings of doom and being overwhelmed, a pounding heart, worry, social phobia, and several panic attacks. I also had hormone imbalances, suffered from terrible premenstrual syndrome (PMS), and had adrenal fatigue. This seemed crazy, as I've always been very adventurous—rock climbing, ice climbing, mountaineering, mountain biking, skiing, and traveling the world.

For me, this situation was due to stress and overwork, combined with a diet that seemed healthy but didn't include any animal protein. On top of this, I have a genetic predisposition to blood sugar issues and food sensitivities, and a greater than average need for zinc and vitamin B_6. I say "for me" because each person is biochemically unique; we all have different needs and imbalances.

I am now completely anxiety free, but I had to figure it out myself, the hard way. I started by reading many books, mostly on PMS. *Before the Change: Taking Charge of Your Perimenopause* (1998), by Anne Louise Gittleman, was wonderful and helped me figure out many things, particularly my need for zinc, B_6, magnesium, progesterone, and gamma-linolenic acid (an omega-6 fatty acid), most of which, little did I know, addressed an inherited condition called pyroluria (which I tested for and confirmed years later).

I consulted with a nurse practitioner and a naturopath, worked to reduce the stress in my life, and supported my adrenals with better nutrition. I went back to school to study nutrition, practiced Iyengar yoga regularly, and incorporated the commonsense approach of traditional diets and eating real, whole, good-quality food, including animal protein. I started working as a nutritionist so I could share what I'd learned. All the while, I attended many conferences on nutrition, mental health, and functional medicine (which focuses on prevention and underlying causes, rather than symptoms).

Along the way, I tried to learn as much as I could about optimal physical and mental health, and also had the good fortune to work at the clinic of one of the greatest pioneers in this field, nutritional psychologist Julia Ross. What I learned from Julia, her book *The Mood Cure* (2004), and working with clients at her Recovery Systems Clinic was incredible. Using amino acids and other critical nutrients, as well as dietary changes and biochemical balancing, we helped so many people resolve mood disorders, addictions, cravings, and eating disorders.

I now have my own practice, focused on natural solutions for anxiety and other mood problems using whole foods, nutrients, and lifestyle changes to help my clients be their healthiest, look their best, and feel on top of the world emotionally. Although I work mostly with women, these tools will work for men too.

I've written this book to share what I've learned in my journey, and because the solutions in this book have helped so many people alleviate their anxiety, fear, worry, feelings of impending doom, panic attacks, and social phobia, along with the uncomfortable physical symptoms that accompany anxiety. There are many incredible holistic practitioners, authors, and researchers with experience and expertise in this area. I've done my best to pull from all their expertise, as well as my own knowledge and clinical experience. I want to make it easy for you to find the answers quickly, all in one place, because I'm all too familiar with that awful feeling of anxiety and doom, and I don't want you to have to spend years finding solutions, as I did.

Anxiety Statistics and Facts

According to the Anxiety Disorders Association of America (2010), anxiety disorders are the most prevalent mental illness in the United States, "affecting 40 million adults age 18 and older," or about 18 percent of the U.S. population. The true number is probably higher, as people who don't seek help or who seek only natural solutions aren't included in the count. And adult rates of anxiety are increasing. From the early 1990s to the early 2000s, generalized anxiety disorder tripled, and panic disorder doubled (Skaer, Sclar, and Robison 2008). Other Western countries with lifestyle and eating habits similar to those in the United States have similar levels of anxiety. For example, about 10 percent of Australians will be affected by anxiety disorders at some point in their lives

(Andrews et al. 1999). Many people with anxiety also suffer from related disorders, including depression, bipolar disorder, irritable bowel syndrome, eating and sleep disorders, and substance abuse.

There are various types of anxiety disorders (Anxiety Disorders Association of America 2010):

- **Generalized anxiety disorder (GAD):** persistent, excessive, and unrealistic worry, tension, and anxiety about everyday things

- **Panic disorder:** panic attacks that seem to arise out of the blue, along with preoccupation with and fear of a recurring attack

- **Social anxiety disorder:** anxiety and fear in social situations

- **Specific phobias:** often irrational fears and anxiety about common, usually harmless things, such as insects, heights, thunder, driving, flying, and so on

- **Obsessive-compulsive disorder (OCD):** unwanted and intrusive thoughts that compel the person to engage in ritualistic behaviors in an effort to ease anxiety

- **Post-traumatic stress disorder (PTSD):** anxiety as a result of a life-threatening event, such as war, rape, or a natural disaster

Women are twice as likely as men to be affected by GAD, panic disorder, specific phobias, and PTSD.

This book can help anyone with the symptoms of GAD, panic disorder, social anxiety disorder, or specific phobia. Those with symptoms of OCD or PTSD may benefit too. This book can also help even if you don't have a full-blown anxiety disorder. It's for anyone who experiences anxiety, nervousness, tension, worry, panic, or fear on a regular basis. If you're anxious about some life event, like a job loss or relationship issue, you still need to work on finding a practical solution, but being in good shape nutritionally will help you cope better. One proviso applies to all readers: If you have serious mood problems, are taking medications, or are pregnant or breastfeeding, consult with a professional about following the guidelines in this book.

It's important that you take anxiety and panic attacks seriously, if for no other reason than the stress they place on the heart. Recent research found that women under fifty years of age (Walters et al. 2008) and postmenopausal women (Smoller et al. 2007) who suffer anxiety and panic attacks may have an increased risk of heart disease.

Causes of Anxiety

There are many possible causes of anxiety, from trauma to medication side effects. Many medical conditions also mimic symptoms of anxiety: thyroid disorders and other hormonal imbalances, diabetes, asthma, epilepsy, and heart conditions. I'll briefly touch on hormonal imbalances, but the focus of this book is relieving anxiety through food and the nutrients found in foods, as well as when you eat and other lifestyle habits. In *The Mood Cure*, Julia Ross proposes that "much of our increasing emotional distress stems from easily correctable malfunctions in our brain and body chemistry— malfunctions that are primarily the result of critical, unmet nutritional needs" (2004, 3). The steps outlined in this book will help you correct the malfunctions and imbalances that cause your anxiety.

What Is a Natural Approach and Why Use It?

Improved nutrition, lifestyle changes, exercise, stress reduction techniques, supplements, and mind-body practices are all part of a natural approach to anxiety and other mood problems. James Lake, integrative psychiatrist and author of *Textbook of Integrative Mental Health* (2007), supports these methods for mild to moderate mental health symptoms, as do many other holistic practitioners and researchers.

Why use a natural approach? Perhaps you already feel strongly about taking a natural approach to health whenever possible and want to learn more. Or maybe your anxiety was so severe and you were so desperate that you turned to medications, but now they aren't working as well or as expected, or perhaps they do help but you don't like some of the side effects. Perhaps you know deep down that addressing the root cause is the way to go. Whatever the reason, if you're looking for natural options for combating anxiety, you've come to the right place.

Using natural approaches in the form of foods and nutrients can address the root cause of your anxiety, alleviate symptoms, and keep them from returning. For example, if your anxiety is due to a vitamin B_6 deficiency, it makes the most sense to boost your levels of vitamin B_6. This will also help raise your levels of serotonin, which could improve your mood, sleep, cravings, and, for women, PMS symptoms. It would also be important to look at why your vitamin B_6 is low to start with. Maybe you aren't getting enough in your diet, aren't digesting well, are under a great deal of stress, or have depleted levels from taking birth control pills. This is just one example of a nutrient deficiency that can contribute to anxiety. We'll be looking at this and many others throughout the book.

Good-quality food is the number one priority. Taking supplemental nutrients to correct imbalances is ideally a short-term approach. The exceptions would be if you have an inherited tendency to low levels of some nutrients, or you can't or won't take steps to ease high levels of stress.

It's also important to remember that we are all unique, with individual biochemistry, imbalances, and life circumstances. There isn't a one-size-fits-all magic solution, even among natural approaches. So read each chapter, fill out the questionnaires, and use that information to help you determine which approaches may apply to you.

Overview of the Book

This book is all about how to correct your anxiety-prone biochemistry naturally—starting with changes in your eating habits (chapter 1). You'll also learn when to eat, why you must avoid sugar (and how to reduce your cravings), and how these factors relate to blood sugar issues (chapter 2). You'll learn about the problems associated with caffeine, alcohol, and nicotine (chapter 3), and gluten and other potentially problematic foods (chapter 4). You'll learn about how good digestive function can help with anxiety (chapter 5). Calming amino acids will be covered in the chapter on brain chemistry (chapter 6), and zinc and vitamin B_6 will be covered in the chapter on pyroluria (chapter 7). I'll briefly discuss other beneficial nutrients, such as magnesium, the B vitamins, vitamin D, and inositol, and also touch on other areas that are beyond the scope of nutrition but are integral to a natural approach and may be relevant to you, including hormone imbalances, medication side effects, exposure to toxins, and, last but not least, lifestyle factors, such as exercise, sleep, and relaxation (chapter 8).

I've also created a website for this book (www.antianxietyfood solution.com), where you'll find new research results, additional case studies, an index, summary checklists for each chapter, and additional resources. Be sure to check it from time to time, as I'll continue to post new information as it becomes available.

You'll be able to do much of what I recommend in the book on your own, especially the food and lifestyle changes. You may ultimately find it helpful to work with a nutritionist or a health care provider trained in nutrition, for guidance, support, additional resources, and referrals (for example, for testing).

In addition to addressing your anxiety, your work with this book will probably also lead to improvements in symptoms that you hadn't thought of as being related to your anxiety, such as mood, sleep, and cravings. For example, if your anxiety is related to low levels of serotonin, you should also feel more upbeat and optimistic, experience less irritability and anger, have better self-esteem, and, for women, be free of PMS. You'll also start to sleep better and experience fewer food cravings. By eating better, reducing stress, and addressing any nutritional imbalances, you'll also see an overall improvement in your general health and well-being. With all of this to look forward to, I'm sure you're eager to get started, so turn the page and read on.

CHAPTER 1

Figure Out Your Optimum Antianxiety Diet

Eating real, whole, good-quality food is the foundation of this book and any program to prevent and alleviate mental health issues such as anxiety, obsessive tendencies, worry, panic attacks, and depression, as well as to maintain optimal mental health. This approach, combined with eating according to your own unique needs, will help calm your anxious mind.

Although there is much clinical evidence for the benefits of eating this way, food and its effects on mental health have not been studied a great deal until recently. However, recent studies have shed more light on the importance of diet. I'm thrilled and anticipate more interest in this area of research. An Australian study looking at both anxiety and depression among women found a link between better diet quality and better mental health (Jacka, Pasco, Mykletun, Williams, Hodge, et al. 2010). Among the participants, those who ate a whole foods diet of vegetables, fruit, fish, whole grains, and grass-fed lean red meat and lamb had a lower likelihood of both anxiety and depression. The researchers referred to this as a "traditional" diet. Those who ate a typical Western diet, replete with processed, refined, fried, and sugary foods and beer, were more likely to experience depression. There was also a tenuous relationship between depression and what the researchers referred to as a "modern" diet of fruit, salads, fish, tofu, beans, nuts, yogurt, and red wine. However, the authors proposed that this may be due to women attempting to improve their mental health by improving their diets, since this sort of diet was more often consumed by younger and more educated women.

Other recent food studies have focused on depression, and results indicate that there's a strong link between good mental health and eating real, whole foods. This very likely has a bearing on anxiety, as anxiety often co-occurs with depression and there are often common underlying biochemical mechanisms in both. For example, a recent British study of 3,486 middle-aged men and women compared those eating a Mediterranean-style, whole foods diet, plentiful in vegetables, fruit, and fish, to those who ate a diet high in processed foods, sweetened desserts, fried foods, processed meat, refined grains, and high-fat dairy products (Akbaraly et al. 2009). Those who ate a diet high in processed foods had a higher risk of depression five years later. Another recent study (Sanchez-Villegas et al. 2009), which looked at over ten thousand Spanish adults, found that those who consumed a Mediterranean diet similar to that in the British study, along with moderate amounts of alcohol, were less prone to depressive disorders.

An editorial in the *American Journal of Psychiatry* offered a very powerful comment on the three food and mood studies outlined previously: "It is both compelling and daunting to consider that dietary intervention at an individual or population level could reduce rates of psychiatric disorders. There are exciting implications for clinical care, public health, and research" (Freeman 2010, 245).

An even more recent study (Jacka, Pasco, Mykletun, Williams, Nicholson, et al. 2010), paralleling the earlier Australian study on diet, depression, and anxiety, found that women who ate a quality whole foods diet were less likely to have bipolar disorder. An added benefit is that eating real, whole, good-quality foods also helps prevent a variety of physical issues, including high blood pressure, irritable bowel syndrome, cancer, heart disease, and arthritis.

I encourage you to start with one of the antianxiety diets explained next, and then keep building on your knowledge and refining your choices as you continue reading this book. Bring a spirit of exploration to how you eat, learning new recipes and food preparation techniques, trying new foods, and finding enjoyment in shopping, cooking, and eating. All the while, pay close attention to how you feel when you eat or exclude particular foods. If you simply start eating real, whole, good-quality foods, you'll notice how much better you start to feel moodwise, and you'll probably start to sleep better and have fewer cravings. It really is that simple! Remember, real food is the foundation and everything else in this book builds on this foundation.

For many people, just making food changes is enough to eliminate anxiety. I had one client with anxiety, moodiness, and very poor-quality sleep who saw a huge improvement after simply switching from eating fast foods once a day to eating real foods, eating regularly (including eating breakfast), and getting enough protein, especially at breakfast.

The Antianxiety Food Solution Diets

Based on my experience, there is no single antianxiety food solution that works for everyone. We all have distinctive nutritional needs, sometimes referred to as biochemical individuality. This means there's no one-size fits-all approach—for diet, exercise, nutritional supplements, or medications. Determining and meeting your unique nutritional needs is key in overcoming anxiety, and most mental and physical health problems.

This section provides an overview of four antianxiety diets that I've found to be effective, with details on all the foods to include and avoid, as well as bonus foods you can try later, once you've established a good foundation for your own antianxiety diet. Some trial and error is involved in finding the optimal diet for you. The progression I outline next provides a methodical approach that will help you determine whether you have various common food sensitivities that could be contributing to your anxiety.

I'll discuss the specifics of what to include and what to avoid in the remainder of this chapter, and then cover some important topics in greater detail in other chapters: avoiding sugar (chapter 2) and caffeine (chapter 3), how to assess for any food sensitivities (chapter 4), and how to get the most from the food you eat by improving your digestion (chapter 5). Taking various supplements based on your individual needs is discussed throughout the rest of the book where relevant.

Antianxiety Food Solution Diets	Diet 1: Gluten free	Diet 2: Gluten free, dairy free	Diet 3: Grain free, dairy free	Diet 4: Traditional foods
What to Include				
Eat **real, whole, good-quality foods**, preferably organic	okay	okay	okay	okay
Eat **frequently enough** for blood sugar stability	okay	okay	okay	okay
Eat **quality animal protein**, such as grass-fed meat, wild game, pastured poultry and eggs, and wild fish	okay	okay	okay	okay
Eat **nonstarchy fresh vegetables**, such as cauliflower, broccoli, and green, leafy vegetables	okay	okay	okay	okay
Eat **fresh fruit**, such as berries, apples, oranges, and peaches	okay	okay	okay	okay
Eat **good fats** from olive oil, butter, coconut oil, avocados, nuts, and seeds	okay	okay	okay	okay
Keep hydrated with water, herbal teas, and fresh vegetable juices	okay	okay	okay	okay
Eat **legumes**, such as lentils, chickpeas, and black beans	okay	okay		okay
Eat **starchy fresh vegetables**, such as potatoes, sweet potatoes, and winter squash	okay	okay		okay
Eat **gluten-free whole grains**, such as brown rice, corn, quinoa, millet, and amaranth	okay	okay		okay

Antianxiety Food Solution Diets	Diet 1: Gluten free	Diet 2: Gluten free, dairy free	Diet 3: Grain free, dairy free	Diet 4: Traditional foods
Consume dairy, such as milk, cheese, yogurt, and kefir	okay			okay
Eat whole grains that contain gluten, such as wheat, rye, and barley				okay
What to Avoid				
Avoid grains that contain gluten, such as wheat, rye, and barley	avoid	avoid	avoid	
Avoid dairy		avoid	avoid	
Avoid all grains, starchy vegetables, and legumes			avoid	
Avoid empty foods, such as bad fats, processed foods (especially those with artificial ingredients), genetically modified foods, caffeine, and sugar, artificial sweeteners, and sodas	avoid	avoid	avoid	avoid
What to Try Later				
Eat bonus foods, such as organ meats, fermented foods, broths, and fresh herbs	okay	okay	okay	okay

Antianxiety Food Solution Diet 1: Gluten Free

I recommend starting with a gluten-free diet, and I typically have my clients begin with this approach. Eat this way for two weeks and then reintroduce gluten, following the instructions for a gluten elimination-challenge trial as described in chapter 4. If you already know you don't tolerate gluten well, there's obviously no need to reintroduce it. This diet is also advocated by Julia Ross in both *The Mood Cure* (2004) and *The Diet Cure* (2011).

Antianxiety Food Solution Diet 2: Gluten Free and Dairy Free

If you try the previous diet for a few weeks and still have problems that seem to be diet related, eliminate dairy for two weeks and then reintroduce it, again as described in chapter 4. Dairy is the next food group to be removed because it's a common food allergen, and also commonly a problem for people who are sensitive to gluten. If you already know you don't tolerate dairy well, there's obviously no need to reintroduce it, and you can begin with this diet, rather than a solely gluten-free diet. This is a modified version of the first diet.

Antianxiety Food Solution Diet 3: Grain Free and Dairy Free

If you try the second diet for a few weeks and still have anxiety and other mood issues, low energy, or sleep and digestive issues, try the third diet, which is the most restrictive. This diet is completely free of all grains (including gluten-free grains) and dairy, and also free of starchy vegetables and legumes. This is a modified version of the Paleolithic diet proposed by Loren Cordain in *The Paleo Diet* (2001) and the approach advocated by Natasha Campbell-McBride in *Gut and Psychology Syndrome* (2008).

Antianxiety Food Solution Diet 4: Traditional Foods

If you're following any of the previous diets and find you're doing well and free of anxiety, you can experiment with a traditional foods approach, which is the least restrictive and includes, among other things, fermented grains and raw dairy. Of course, if you have celiac disease, food allergies, or food sensitivities (discussed in chapter 4), continue to exclude the foods you have difficulty with. The traditional foods diet is a modified version of the approach proposed by Sally Fallon in *Nourishing Traditions* (2001).

Foods to Include

Once you've decided which diet you'll start with, use the preceding table to figure out which foods are included and then follow the guidelines in the next sections. Bear in mind that the diets outlined previously are somewhat generic. Depending on your unique needs, certain foods, categories of food, or approaches may be better for you than others. Experiment to find what works best for you, and feel free to mix and match. For example, you may find you feel best mostly adhering to the third diet and eating no grains, yet you tolerate some forms of dairy, such as yogurt. With all four diets, you may need to reduce or totally eliminate fruit for a short time if candida is an issue (see chapter 5).

While you're figuring out what diet is best for you, keep a detailed food log (appendix 2) to help you determine how different foods may be affecting you. Also, be aware that when I work with clients, we typically address many of the other areas covered in this book alongside a basic dietary approach. So as you begin to experiment with the antianxiety diets, I encourage you to read ahead and make other changes that seem appropriate to your situation. However, if this starts to get overwhelming and you feel more anxious, just implement the solutions in a way that works for you, even if that means taking baby steps and making just one or two changes at a time. If you go that route, I suggest using what I call "eating levels of sophistication," a step-by-step approach that will slowly but surely transition you away from a typical Western diet, sometimes called the standard American diet (SAD):

1. Avoid sugar, foods containing sugar, and "white foods" (white flour, white rice, white pasta, and other refined grains).

2. Avoid all boxed and processed foods and all foods containing artificial colors and other additives.

3. Avoid foods that you're sensitive to or that commonly cause problems, such as wheat (even whole or sprouted wheat).

4. Include more high-quality vegetables, fruit, and protein.

5. Be sure to eat breakfast (including some protein) and healthy snacks.

6. Switch to all or mostly organic foods and start to experiment with the bonus foods discussed later in this chapter.

7. For protein, switch to grass-fed meat, pastured poultry and eggs, and wild fish.

8. Eat fermented foods, soaked grains (if you tolerate grains), organ meats, and broths regularly.

9. Whenever possible, eat local and seasonal foods.

Eat Real, Whole, Good-Quality Foods

Real, whole, traditional, and unrefined foods are nutrient dense and as close to their natural state as possible. They come from nature, not a package, and are ideally local and in season, and preferably organic. It may be the way you ate as a child (if you were fortunate, as I was), or perhaps it's how your grandparents ate. Most real food is fresh and perishable, and doesn't have a long shelf life. You'll find these foods in your garden, on traditional (not agribusiness) farms, at farmers' markets and food co-ops, at fish markets or in the ocean, and on the perimeters of the supermarket. They haven't been processed, manufactured, or packaged. They shouldn't have labels, and if they do, they shouldn't read like a chemistry experiment; the ingredients should be recognizable as real foods. Some examples are home-cooked vegetable soup instead of instant or canned vegetable soup, fresh cream instead of nondairy creamer, and home-cooked meat, rice, and fresh vegetables instead of a TV dinner.

A diet based on real, whole food truly does serve as the foundation for ending anxiety, providing key nutrients that are essential for the body's production of neurotransmitters and hormones. It is the synergistic combination of nutrients that is an antianxiety powerhouse: amino acids from proteins (such as eggs), the mineral zinc from red meat, the mineral magnesium from leafy, green vegetables, B vitamins from grains, omega-3 fatty acids from fish and meat, antioxidants from vegetables and fruit—and more. You really are what you eat. Hippocrates, the father of Western medicine, took that a step further, saying, "Let food be your medicine and your medicine be your food." More recently, orthomolecular psychiatrist Abram Hoffer made a similar point: "Physical and mental diseases are affected by what we put into our mouths—or fail to take in as nourishment" (Hoffer and Walker 1996, 204). The orthomolecular concept is simple: use optimal nutrition to heal and prevent disease and dysfunction, including anxiety.

Given that the food you eat is your fuel, quality is very important. Whenever possible, opt for choices that are organic, grass-fed, wild, pastured, and free of pesticides, hormones, and antibiotics. Red meat should be from animals that were grass-fed. Dairy products should come from cows, goats, or sheep raised in a similar way. For poultry and eggs, the ideal is pastured, meaning the birds forage in a pasture and aren't fed grain exclusively. In addition to being of better quality for our consumption, animals raised this way are also more humanely treated. Fish should be wild, not farmed, and produce should be organic or pesticide free, and preferably locally grown. Although I don't repeat this point throughout the book, eating real, whole, good-quality food is the foundation of any holistic approach for anxiety.

Eat Frequently Enough

While what you eat makes a huge difference with anxiety, when you eat can also be key. Skipping breakfast and not eating frequently enough during the day can result in low blood sugar, with symptoms including anxiety, nervousness, and irritability (Harp and Fox 1990). Following the guidelines in chapter 2, typically makes a huge difference. For now, I'll just say be sure to eat breakfast (with a good-quality protein source, such as eggs), eat three meals and at least two healthful snacks daily, and include carbohydrates, protein, and fats in all of your meals and most of your snacks.

Eat Quality Animal Protein

Although protein is also found in dairy and to a lesser extent in legumes, grains, nuts, and seeds, the most concentrated forms (and in my experience the most beneficial for mental health) are meat, poultry, eggs, and fish. Protein contains amino acids, and the protein you eat directly affects levels of amino acids in your blood and brain, which in turn affects levels of neurotransmitters that play a role in mood (Fernstrom 1981). This topic is discussed in detail in chapter 7.

If you are a vegetarian, I respect your personal choice in this matter, but I highly encourage you to be open to the possibility of trying animal protein. If you see benefits, as many of my formerly vegetarian clients with anxiety and depression do, then you'll know that this could play an important role in helping you overcome anxiety. If you're initially unwilling or unable to eat meat, don't despair. Consider these sources of protein: legumes, nuts, sprouts, hemp, dairy, and fermented or sprouted soy products like tempeh and tofu. Do this in conjunction with the dietary guidelines in this chapter, and make sure you don't rely heavily on processed soy products. Also consider supplementing with whey, pea, or rice protein powder; a free-form amino acid blend; additional iron, zinc, omega-3 fatty acids and B_{12}, if needed. And if you continue to have unresolved mood problems despite implementing the other suggestions in this book, please reassess and consider incorporating eggs and possibly fish into your diet, and then meat if you're willing to go that far. If it's any consolation, I, too, was a vegetarian before I discovered the dietary factors involved in my anxiety, and I really do relate to your ethical concerns. However, based on my personal and clinical experience, I am no longer a fan of vegetarian and vegan diets, especially for those with mental health issues.

Red Meat

All of your animal protein should be free of antibiotics and hormones. With regard to red meat, the best quality is grass fed, and the Australian study mentioned at the beginning of this chapter (Jacka, Pasco, Mykletun, Williams, Hodge, et al. 2010) found that including grass-fed red meat in the diet had mental health benefits. In fact, in an interview in January 2010, the lead researcher in that study, Dr. Felice Jacka, stated, "We've traditionally thought of omega-3s as only coming from fatty fish, but actually good-quality red meat, that is, naturally raised [meaning grass fed] has very good levels of omega-3 fatty acids, whereas red meat that comes from feedlots tends to be higher in omega-6 fatty acids—a fatty acid profile that is far less healthy and may in fact be associated with more mental health problems" (Cassels 2010). Via e-mail correspondence, Dr. Jacka informed me that "consumption of beef and lamb was inversely associated with depression.... Those eating less of this form of red meat were more likely to be depressed." Again, with the anxiety-depression link, and based on my clinical experience, eating red meat is also highly likely to benefit you if you have anxiety.

Meat from grass-fed cattle also contains more conjugated linoleic acids (CLAs), vitamin E, vitamin C, glutathione, and beta-carotene than grain-fed cattle (Daley et al. 2010)—all nutrients that help protect against cancer. In addition, red meat is a great source of vitamins B_6, B_{12}, and D, and minerals that are important for mood, including zinc, iron, and selenium. For some people, zinc and vitamin B_6 deficiency plays a key role in anxiety disorders (see chapter 8), and red meat can be a good source of both of these nutrients.

You may have concerns related to consuming red meat. However, recent studies suggest that there isn't enough evidence to support a positive association between consumption of red meat (and fat) and colorectal cancer (Alexander and Cushing 2010) or ovarian cancer (Kolahdooz et al. 2010)—and that the quality of the meat may be more of an issue, with processed meats being a likely culprit (ibid; Micha, Wallace, and Mozaffarian 2010). Another recent study failed to find an association between meat consumption and risk of stroke (Preis et al. 2010). Finally, some reviews actually suggest that moderate consumption of lean red meat, and grass-fed beef in particular, is actually beneficial for heart health and overall health, and helps protect against cancer (Daley et al. 2010).

For the best-quality meat, buy from farmers' markets or local farmers if possible. If you can't find grass-fed meat locally and you're willing to purchase it online, check out U.S. Wellness Meats (see resources). They offer a great selection of good-quality grass-fed meat products (and poultry).

Poultry and Eggs

Poultry is an excellent source of amino acids, especially tryptophan, and the B vitamin niacin, and a good source of vitamin B_6 and selenium. Chickens foraging in a pasture have higher levels of omega-3 fatty acids than grain-fed chicken, so pastured chickens are best both for consumption and as a source of eggs. The next best choice is organic.

Like red meat, eggs also have a bad reputation, and many people ask me if it's okay to eat eggs, particularly egg yolks. Eggs truly are healthful and an important part of a diet based on real, whole foods, and recent research indicates that they don't actually contribute to heart disease (Jones 2009; Ruxton 2010). Eggs are a great source of affordable high-quality protein and contain selenium, iodine, and vitamins A and D. The yolk is a wonderful source of choline, which is very important for brain health. Choline is a component of lecithin, a group of substances in the yolk that actually helps with fat digestion. However, eggs are one of the common causes of food sensitivity (discussed in chapter 4), so keep this in mind. Also, be aware that to get 20 to 30 grams of protein, a good serving size of protein for a meal, you need to eat three medium-sized eggs.

Fish and Other Seafood

Seafood is a great source of amino acids, omega-3 fatty acids, zinc, iodine, iron, calcium, selenium, and vitamins B_{12}, A, and D, many of which are beneficial for mood disorders. Again, for some people zinc deficiency plays a key role in anxiety disorders (see chapter 8), so seafood can be helpful. Oysters have particularly high levels of zinc, and mussels, clams, and crab have good levels as well.

The Australian, Spanish, and British studies discussed at the beginning of the chapter (Jacka, Pasco, Mykletun, Williams, Hodge, et al. 2010; Jacka, Pasco, Mykletun, Williams, Nicholson, et al. 2010; Sanchez-Villegas et al. 2009; Akbaraly et al. 2009) all found that including fish in the diet improved mental health. Another study (Tanskanen et al. 2001) found that the prevalence of depression was lower in countries where consumption of seafood is high. Given the link between anxiety and depression, it's possible that seafood consumption could also help reduce the incidence of anxiety. Many studies have looked at how supplementing with omega-3 fish oils affects mental health. Some have shown mood improvements (for example, Haag 2003), while others have shown no real benefits (for example, Stahl et al. 2008). My recommendation is that you eat fish, including some oily fish, such as salmon or sardines, and only supplement with fish oil if you know for sure you have low levels of omega-3s. (See chapter 8 for more on essential fatty acids.)

As always, quality is important. Wild fish is the best choice, in part because farmed fish contains antibiotics and artificial colors. In addition, one animal study found a link between farmed fish and increased risk of diabetes (Ruzzin et al. 2010). Among wild ocean fish, Pacific halibut and cod are good choices; in terms of fresh-water fish, trout is a good choice. Do eat some oily fish, such as Alaskan salmon, sablefish, sardines, and pilchards, as they contain excellent levels of omega-3 fatty acids. Sardines may be an acquired taste, but they really are great, and they're also very affordable and easy to take with you when you travel. Although I generally recommend against canned foods, I do think they're a good option when it comes to salmon, sardines, mussels, oysters, and, occasionally, tuna. One caveat in regard to tuna: eat it in moderation or make sure you purchase from a source that tests mercury levels. And in general, select fish canned in olive oil or water, not cottonseed oil, and make sure that any shellfish you purchase are harvested from clean, wild waters, since they tend to accumulate toxins.

Much research confirms that the many benefits of eating fish (in moderation) outweigh some of the risks of toxicity, and there is some evidence that the selenium that naturally occurs in certain fish and shellfish may offer protection from mercury toxicity (Ralston and Raymond 2010). Smaller wild fish are the best choice because mercury and polychlorinated biphenyls (PCBs) build up in farmed fish, shellfish, and larger fish, such as swordfish, shark, and California halibut. It's best to avoid these, and especially important for children, pregnant and breastfeeding women, and anyone with health problems, physical or mental. Since you're reading this book to help with your anxiety, that list includes you.

For good information on safe and environmentally sound seafood, visit the website of the Monterey Bay Aquarium (see resources). If you're fortunate enough to be near the ocean, buy fresh fish from fish markets. Otherwise, purchase fresh or frozen fish from your local store. If you're willing to purchase seafood online, Vital Choice (see resources) is a great source of good-quality seafood.

Sources of animal protein: Red meat (such as beef, lamb, bison, and wild game) from grass-fed animals, poultry and eggs from pastured birds, wild fish (such as sole, salmon, sardines, and pilchards) and other seafood (such as shrimp, mussels, and oysters), and whey protein powder (although derived from dairy and, strictly speaking, not a real, whole food, whey is included here because it's a concentrated source of high-quality protein).

How much to eat: Eat a 3- to 4-ounce serving of quality protein three times a day. Each 3- to 4-ounce serving is a palm-sized portion and provides 20 to 30 grams of protein. Three eggs is equivalent to one protein serving providing 20 to 30 grams of protein. A serving of whey should be 20 to 30 grams of protein. Eat fish two or three times a week.

Eat Nonstarchy Fresh Vegetables

Vegetables are an important part of the whole foods diets that proved so beneficial for mood in the four food studies mentioned throughout this chapter (Jacka, Pasco, Mykletun, Williams, Hodge, et al. 2010; Jacka, Pasco, Mykletun, Williams, Nicholson, et al. 2010; Sanchez-Villegas et al. 2009; Akbaraly et al. 2009). They provide minerals, such as calcium, magnesium, manganese, potassium, and zinc; many of the B vitamins; and antioxidants, such as vitamins A, C, E, and K. Many of these nutrients play an important role in mood and emotional well-being. In addition, the antioxidants in vegetables (and fruits) provide protection against increased oxidative stress, a physiological condition characterized by excessive levels of free radicals that's often associated with mood disorders (Tsaluchidu et al. 2008). It's best not to boil vegetables, as this leaches out many of these nutrients. If you do boil vegetables, try to use the water in a soup, sauce, or broth.

Fresh local or homegrown produce that's organic or pesticide free is typically more nutrient dense and often tastes better (Davis 2009). An added bonus is that eating this way is also beneficial for the earth, as it doesn't introduce synthetic chemicals into the environment. Studies of farmworkers have shown a link between pesticide exposure and cognitive and psychological problems, including anxiety and depression (Mearns, Dunn, and Lees-Haley 1994). More recently, a study found that even low levels of pesticides in conventionally grown vegetables and fruit increased children's risk of developing attention deficit/hyperactivity disorder (Bouchard et al. 2010). Hopefully more studies will examine the impacts of pesticides on the nervous system.

The Environmental Working Group, a nonprofit organization dedicated to protecting public health and the environment, regularly issues a shopper's guide to the "dirty dozen" and the "clean fifteen" (2010). The "dirty dozen" are fruits and vegetables grown conventionally that are mostly likely to be contaminated with pesticides; the "clean fifteen" are those least likely to be contaminated. Organic is always a better choice for your health and the environment, and this is especially the case when purchasing the "dirty dozen": apples, bell peppers, blueberries, celery, cherries, grapes, kale or collard greens, nectarines, peaches, potatoes, spinach, and strawberries.

Because the "clean fifteen" are lowest in pesticides, they don't necessarily have to be organic: asparagus, avocados, cabbage, cantaloupe, eggplant, grapefruit, honeydew, kiwi, mangoes, onions, pineapple, sweet corn, sweet peas, sweet potatoes, and watermelon.

Nonstarchy fresh vegetables: Artichokes, asparagus, avocados, bell peppers, bok choy, burdock, carrots, celery, cilantro, cruciferous vegetables (such as broccoli, Brussels sprouts, cabbage, and cauliflower), cucumber, daikon, eggplant, fennel, garlic, ginger, green beans, green leafy vegetables and salad greens (such as arugula, beet greens, chard, collard greens, kale, lettuce, mixed baby greens, mustard greens, nettles, and spinach), mushrooms, onions, parsley, radishes, sweet peas, summer squash (such as crookneck squash, pattypans, and zucchini), tomatoes, turnips, and water chestnuts.

How much to eat: Aim for at least four and preferably more servings of nonstarchy vegetables a day. A serving is about 1 cup for cooked vegetables, or double that for raw leafy greens and salads.

Eat Fresh Fruit

Fruits are also an important part of the whole foods diets that had proven benefits for mood (Jacka, Pasco, Mykletun, Williams, Hodge, et al. 2010; Jacka, Pasco, Mykletun, Williams, Nicholson, et al. 2010; Sanchez-Villegas et al. 2009; Akbaraly et al. 2009). They provide similar nutritional benefits as vegetables, as explained previously, and also come with the same concerns about pesticides, so be sure to follow the Environmental Working Group's recommendations in regard to the "dirty dozen" and "clean fifteen."

Fresh fruit: Apples, apricots, bananas, blackberries, blueberries, cantaloupe, cherries, cranberries, figs, grapefruit, grapes, honeydew, kiwi, lemons, mangoes, melons, nectarines, oranges, papayas, peaches, pears, pineapple, plums, raspberries, strawberries, tangerines, and watermelon.

How much to eat: Two to four servings daily (less of the higher-sugar tropical fruits). A serving is typically equivalent to about one small apple or ½ cup of berries. And remember, you may have to reduce or totally eliminate fruit for a short time if candida is an issue.

Eat Good Fats

For several decades, dietary fat has had a bad reputation, but this is undeserved. Fats are key for the nervous system, hormonal health, and many physiological processes. So you really do need good fats and shouldn't try to avoid or restrict them.

Many studies support the emotional and physical benefits of consuming adequate amounts of good fats. In a study comparing a group deriving 41 percent of their calories from fat with a group getting 25 percent of their calories from fat, the group eating more fat had less anxiety, less anger, and better overall mood—with no appreciable differences in total cholesterol, LDL (so-called bad cholesterol), or triglycerides (Wells et al. 1998). One review of the relationship between dietary fats and heart disease (Ramsden et al. 2009) found that the quality of fats was more important than the quantity. The authors of that study propose trans fats and vegetable-based fats are problematic, whereas saturated fats (including coconut oil) aren't a risk factor in heart disease. Olive oil, an important component of the Mediterranean diet and widely recognized for its many health benefits, helped reduce anxiety in a recent animal study (Pitozzi et al. 2010). Another important reason to include sufficient dietary fats is that they help the body absorb carotenoids (such as beta-carotene) from salad greens and vegetables (Brown et al. 2004). Joseph Pizzorno, a prominent naturopathic physician, discusses the effectiveness of flaxseed oil in helping patients with agoraphobia (fear of having a panic attack in an inescapable situation or a situation where this would be embarrassing; this frequently manifests as avoidance of open spaces, public places, and crowds) and signs of fatty acid deficiency, such as dry skin, dandruff, brittle fingernails, and nerve disorders (Pizzorno and Murray 2000).

Because so many people have aimed to cut fat from their diets in recent decades, you may need a little extra help here, so I'll offer a few tips on how to incorporate more good fats into your diet. Try adding full-fat coconut milk to a smoothie, use it in the sauce for a Thai curry, pour it over fruit as a dessert, or blend it with fresh fruit and then freeze it to make ice pops. You can buy fresh coconut, but for convenience you may want to use canned coconut milk (often found in the Asian section of supermarkets), coconut butter and oil (available in natural food stores), and unsweetened dried coconut. Coconut oil (like butter) can withstand higher cooking temperatures than other oils, including olive oil, so it's great to cook with.

Olive oil is great to enjoy on salads and vegetables to enhance absorption of their nutrients. Olive oil and vinegar or freshly squeezed lemon juice make a nice salad dressing, and plain olive oil is also wonderful over cooked whole grains. When shopping, make sure that the olive oil and any other oils you purchase are cold pressed and organic, and sold in a dark bottle.

Because butter is a saturated fat, it's good for higher-heat cooking, and melted butter is, of course, also wonderful on cooked vegetables. If you have a dairy sensitivity, try ghee (clarified butter); it's free of casein and lactose, the constituents of milk that typically cause problems.

Flaxseed oil, which is less stable than most of the other good fats, shouldn't be used in heated dishes (though you can drizzle it over cooked foods). Store it in the fridge, and make sure it's in an opaque bottle so it isn't damaged by exposure to light. Freshly ground flaxseeds (also to be stored in the fridge) are great in smoothies and on salads.

Avocados are great in salads and dips, as are nuts and seeds. Ideally, nuts should be soaked before you eat them. This neutralizes naturally occurring enzyme inhibitors and aids in digestion and absorption. Pumpkin seeds, which are higher in protein than many other seeds, are a good source of tryptophan, zinc, iron, omega-3 fatty acids, calcium, and B vitamins. After soaking them for about six hours, drain them well and try roasting them with spices, such as sea salt, pepper, turmeric, and ginger. Not only is this a delicious snack, but it also helps control blood sugar levels and is a favorite of mine for mood health. One important note in regard to nuts and seeds: avoid store-bought dry-roasted versions, as they may contain harmful and rancid fats.

Of course, if you follow the other guidelines in this chapter, you'll also be getting some additional beneficial fats (both omega-3s and saturated fats) from meat, poultry, eggs, fish, and dairy. For example, full-fat dairy products, such as Greek yogurt and cottage cheese, provide a good source of fat, as do chicken skin and grass-fed meat. Pemmican, an early convenience food of the Native Americans, is made from ground jerky, animal fat, and cranberries, and it is my favorite high-energy snack "bar."

Good fats: Olives and olive oil, butter or ghee, coconut oil and other coconut products, avocados, flaxseeds and flax oil, other seeds (sunflower seeds, sesame seeds, and pumpkin seeds), nuts (such as almonds, Brazil nuts, cashews, and walnuts), and pemmican.

How much to eat: Eat some form of good fat with each meal and snack. Each day, eat at least ¼ cup (and preferably more) of good fats and about ¼ cup of nuts and seeds, and be aware that you may need more, especially if you're eating fewer starches.

Keep Hydrated

Keep hydrated with at least 2 quarts (64 fluid ounces) of filtered water daily—or more if you're exercising or very active. In addition to plain water, try water with lemon or orange slices or a bit of cranberry juice, or drink herbal caffeine-free teas, such as mint, chamomile, lemon-ginger, licorice, and orange. Other good beverage options include broths, coconut water, freshly squeezed vegetable juices, and fermented beverages like kombucha (a fermented tea) or water kefir (all of the benefits of regular kefir, but without the dairy!). Drinking a cup of hot water (plain or with a bit of fresh lemon juice or ginger) first thing in the morning is not only tasty

26

and stimulating, it's also an Ayurvedic remedy for digestive and liver support.

Eat Legumes

Legumes are a good source of both protein and carbohydrates, and are also high in beneficial fiber. However, people have various degrees of difficulty with digesting them. Soaking legumes overnight and then cooking them with sea vegetables, particularly kombu, may improve digestibility. Sprouting is another good option. If you try these methods and still have difficulty with legumes, consider an elimination-challenge trial. Sensitivity is common enough that legumes are excluded from the third antianxiety diet outlined previously, as are starchy vegetables and grains. You'll have to experiment to determine what works for you. (See the information on the GAPS diet in chapter 4 for more on this.)

However, I recommend avoiding processed soy products altogether. Not only is soy a common food allergen, but it's also extremely difficult to digest. In addition, it may depress thyroid function and affect the reproductive system. Even if you tolerate soy, I recommend that you limit your consumption to small amounts of fermented soy in the form of miso and wheat-free tamari, and an occasional serving of organic tofu or tempeh. Doing a soy elimination-challenge trial is always an option if you're uncertain.

Legumes: Black beans, black-eyed peas, garbanzo beans (and hummus), lentils, pinto beans, and split peas, and others.

How much to eat: Unless you need to avoid legumes, aim for up to ½ cup of cooked legumes a few times a week.

Eat Starchy Fresh Vegetables

Although most people tolerate starchy vegetables just fine, for some people they're a problem. That's why they're excluded from the third antianxiety diet. You'll have to experiment and see whether they're okay for you. (Again, see the information on the GAPS diet in chapter 4 for more on this.)

If you can tolerate starchy vegetables, aim for at least one serving a day. They're interchangeable with grains.

In terms of shopping and cooking, many of the same guidelines apply as for nonstarchy vegetables. When possible, choose vegetables that are organic, local, and in season, and steam or bake them rather than boiling (except in dishes like soups and stews, where the cooking liquid is part of the dish). Drizzle with butter or oil to enhance nutrient absorption and reduce their effect on blood sugar.

Starchy fresh vegetables: Beets, corn, peas, potatoes, sweet potatoes, turnips, and winter squash (such as butternut and pumpkin).

How much to eat: Unless you need to avoid nonstarchy vegetables, aim for at least one serving a day. One serving is about 1 cup, cooked.

Eat Gluten-Free Whole Grains

As with legumes and starchy vegetables, most people can tolerate gluten-free whole grains, but a subset of people can't, so they are excluded from the third antianxiety diet, which is totally grain free. You'll have to experiment to determine if you can tolerate them. (Again, see chapter 4 for more on this.)

If you can tolerate gluten-free whole grains, aim for at least one serving a day. They're interchangeable with starchy vegetables and grains with gluten.

Brown rice and wild rice are good sources of fiber and B vitamins. Quinoa is easy to digest, has the highest protein content of any grain, and gives you lots of energy; just be sure to rinse it well before cooking. Quinoa, millet, and amaranth are all cooked similarly to rice, but cook more quickly than most types of whole grain rice. While fresh corn is included in the starchy vegetables category, dried corn is more similar to a grain, and corn tortillas and cornbread can help take the place of other foods if you have a problem with gluten. For all grains, soaking or sprouting improves digestibility. When possible, soak grains for at least eight hours before cooking. For morning oatmeal, soak the oats overnight; they'll cook very quickly the next morning.

Gluten-free whole grains: Amaranth, brown rice (and other whole grain rice), buckwheat, corn, millet, quinoa, and wild rice, preferably soaked or sprouted. Oats are also gluten-free, but if you have celiac disease or a severe gluten sensitivity, be sure to choose certified gluten-free oats due to cross-contamination in processing and transportation.

How much to eat: Aim for at least one serving a day of gluten-free whole grains. One serving is about 1 cup, cooked.

Consume Dairy

Dairy is a good source of protein and fat (provided you avoid fat-free dairy). It's also rich in tryptophan, which has important mood benefits (discussed in chapter 8). Although many people can tolerate dairy, it is one of the most common problematic foods, which explains why it's excluded from two of the antianxiety diets. Because of this, I encourage you to try a two-week dairy elimination-challenge trial even if you don't suspect you have a problem with dairy. That said, a few forms of dairy are less likely to be problematic, particularly whey, ghee (clarified butter), and, for some people, fermented or raw dairy products, or those made from sheep or goat milk.

Fermented dairy products, such as yogurt and kefir, are especially good choices. Not only are they more digestible, but they're also rich in probiotics, or beneficial bacteria. Raw dairy products are often easier to digest than pasteurized and homogenized. However, consuming raw dairy is controversial, so do your own research and consider this carefully to determine what you're comfortable with. Products made with goat or sheep milk may be easier for you to digest than those made with cow's milk. You really have to experiment to find what works for you, so give cottage cheese and hard cheeses a try too. Finally, you may do just fine with dairy as long as you eat it on a rotating basis, meaning that you only eat whatever dairy you can tolerate every three days or so.

Ideally, all dairy products that you consume should come from cows, goats, or sheep that are grass fed and not treated with antibiotics and hormones. The next best choice is organic. If you can't purchase organic dairy products, at least look for those produced without bovine growth hormone.

Dairy: Milk, cheese, yogurt, and kefir from grass-fed cows, sheep, or goats, along with butter, ghee, and whey.

How much to consume: If you tolerate dairy, aim to consume what you can tolerate and consider it part of your protein quota. In regard to whey, you can use 20 to 30 grams mixed into smoothies or other foods.

Eat Whole Grains That Contain Gluten

Given that gluten-containing grains are excluded from three of the four antianxiety diets, gluten-containing grains are really a better fit for the next section of this chapter: "Foods to Avoid." In my experience, gluten consumption and mood issues are often linked, so I encourage you to be cautious here. I recommend you try a two-week gluten elimination-challenge trial, as outlined in chapter 4, even if you don't suspect that it's an issue for you.

If you can tolerate gluten, aim for at least one serving of wheat, rye, or barley a day, keeping in mind that these grains are interchangeable with starchy vegetables and gluten-free grains.

Even if gluten isn't an issue, soaking, sprouting, and fermenting will enhance the digestibility and nutritional value of these grains. So enjoy them in the form of sourdough or sprouted whole grain bread, or crackers made with sprouted grains. And be sure to avoid processed and refined grains and foods made from them, like doughnuts, white bread, and commercial cookies and cakes.

> **Whole grains with gluten:** Whole wheat, rye, and barley, prefer-
> ably soaked, sprouted, or fermented (such as sourdough).
>
> **How much to eat:** If you tolerate gluten, aim for at least one serving
> a day. One serving is about 1 cup, cooked.

Foods to Avoid

Depending on which diet you select and your own unique biochemistry, you'll need to avoid grains that contain gluten, dairy, and
possibly even gluten-free grains, starchy vegetables, or legumes, or
some combination of these foods. Avoiding empty foods is crucial
to all four antianxiety diets.

Gluten, Dairy, and Grains

The rationale for excluding gluten-containing grains (wheat,
rye, and barley) and dairy is that they commonly cause food sensitivities and can give rise to a variety of problems that may have
a bearing on anxiety. Less commonly, all grains are a problem, as
well as starchy vegetables and legumes. As mentioned earlier in this
chapter, you'll have to experiment to determine what works for you.
Chapter 4 discusses this topic in detail and will help you figure this
out.

Avoid Empty Foods

"Empty foods" refers to foods that are devoid of vitality and
lacking in nutrients An additional downside of these foods is that
they often contain harmful substances that may contribute to
anxiety. Some of the empty foods are covered in more detail in
later chapters: various forms of sugar (and artificial sweeteners) in
chapter 2, and caffeine and alcohol in chapter 3. Empty foods don't
have a place in any antianxiety diet—or any other wholesome diet,
for that matter.

Bad fats. Trans fats and hydrogenated oils, produced by industrial processes, are unrecognizable to the body and inherently unhealthful. Avoid them at all costs. Very recently, trans fats have been linked to an increased risk of depression (Sanchez-Villegas 2011). They frequently show up in margarine and a wide variety of processed foods, including coffee creamers and baked goods. And although vegetable oils have been touted as being more healthful, many of them are unstable and therefore unsuitable for dishes that are heated. With the exception of olive oil, I recommend that you steer clear of vegetable oils, such as canola, corn, and soy, and oils that are heat processed and deodorized, as well as commercial salad dressings that contain them. Hopefully you'll adopt an antianxiety diet that doesn't include processed foods, but if you do buy them on occasion, make sure they don't contain any of the bad fats discussed here.

Processed foods. Again, these foods don't have a place in any healthful diet, particularly not in an antianxiety diet. Avoid boxed and packaged foods that contain additives, preservatives, artificial colors, and flavoring agents, such as monosodium glutamate (MSG) and its many variants, including hydrolyzed protein, autolyzed yeast, and sodium caseinate. Common culprits are canned and instant soups, cheese spreads, breakfast cereals, and frozen TV dinners. Also avoid energy bars, which are often loaded with concentrated soy protein and sugar and typically contain wheat. Most canned goods, processed meats, fast food, and condiments fall into this category. Buy real, whole foods instead of processed, and you can't go wrong.

Genetically modified foods. Most of the nonorganic corn, soy, and canola grown in the United States is genetically modified (GM); therefore, any processed food that contains these ingredients is probably a GM food. Why avoid GM foods? At this point, we simply don't know the long-term health consequences. However, preliminary animal studies have shown harmful effects, so concerned researchers are calling for more studies (de Vendômois et al. 2010). Unfortunately, there's no requirement that foods containing GM ingredients be labeled as such, so eating real, whole foods and purchasing organic is the only way to be certain you aren't getting GM foods. For the latest information on GM foods, consult the website of the Institute for Responsible Technology (see resources).

Avoid caffeine. This is covered in detail in chapter 3. In brief, you need to avoid coffee (even decaffeinated), tea (except herbal caffeine-free tea and green tea), possibly chocolate (except dark chocolate), and foods and beverages containing caffeine.

Avoid sugar, artificial sweeteners, and sodas. This is covered in detail in chapter 2. In brief, you need to avoid all forms of added and hidden sugar, such as corn syrup, high-fructose corn syrup, glucose, maltose, and so on; artificial sweeteners such as aspartame, saccharin, and sucralose; sodas and diet sodas; and candies, cakes, and other sweetened baked goods.

Empty foods: Bad fats, processed foods (especially those with artificial additives, preservatives, colors, and flavoring agents), genetically modified foods, caffeine, and sugar, artificial sweeteners or sodas.

How much to eat: None—ever.

Eat Bonus Foods

When I'm working one-on-one with clients, my first objective is to teach them about the basics of eating real whole, good-quality foods, as outlined in this chapter. Once we've determined the basic diet that works for a client, the person usually feels much less anxious. At that point, I introduce the benefits of the bonus foods described next: organ meats, fermented foods, broths, herbs, sprouted beans and seeds, raw apple cider vinegar, sea vegetables, and miso. If any of them appeal to you, feel free to go ahead and include them in your diet. Regarding the others, just keep them in mind for later.

Organ meats. Nutrient dense and very healing, organ meats have been considered a valuable food by many cultures for centuries. Liver is an excellent source of vitamin A, vitamin B_{12}, folic acid, and other B vitamins, and, of course, iron and protein. If you have unfond memories of beef liver, try chicken or lamb liver, as both have a milder flavor. You can also freeze liver, then grate it and add it to dishes like meat loaf. Other options are liver pâté, beef heart, or kidneys. If you're willing to include organ meats, try to eat at least one serving (3-4 ounces) weekly as one of your protein servings.

Fermented foods. Another traditional food with a long and venerable history, fermented foods contain enzymes and probiotics, which help maintain a healthy balance of flora in the gut, supporting digestive health. Some fermented foods are familiar, like yogurt and sauerkraut. Others may seem a bit more exotic, like kefir (including water kefir), kimchi (an Asian pickled vegetable dish), and kombucha (fermented tea). Because of the enormous health benefits of probiotics, more fermented foods are becoming available. You might look for fermented salsa or salad dressings in the refrigerated section of natural food stores, or make your own. Most of these foods are typically eaten in small amounts, like condiments. It's great to include them in your daily diet.

Broths. Homemade bone broths and vegetable broths are incredibly nourishing and rich in minerals. They improve digestion, are very healing for the digestive system, and help boost immunity. Making a bone broth is easy: Fill a large soup pot three-quarters full, then add the bones from a whole chicken (or use beef bones) and 2 tablespoons of apple cider vinegar to help draw the minerals out of the bones. Cover and cook at a low simmer for eight to ten hours for chicken bones, or sixteen to twenty hours for beef bones. Using a slow cooker is another option. Use the broth in stews and soups or to cook brown rice or other whole grains, or just drink it. Try to consume broths a few times week.

Fresh herbs and spices. These make such a difference in the flavor of meals and add immensely to the pleasure of cooking and eating. They also have many medicinal benefits, such as improving digestion (mint and ginger) and helping prevent cancer (turmeric and rosemary). Use garlic, ginger, parsley, and cilantro liberally. Fresh herbs are best, but dried herbs are also fine. I also advocate including high-quality unrefined salt, such as Celtic sea salt or Himalayan salt, in your diet—up to 1 teaspoon daily. It adds to the flavor of meals while also providing important trace minerals, aiding digestion, and whetting the appetite.

Sprouted beans and seeds. These are incredibly nutrient dense, a great source of enzymes, and a relatively good source of vegetable protein. It's easy to grow your own sprouts, especially alfalfa, mung beans, lentils, and broccoli. Try them on salads, or add them to stir-fries right at the end of cooking.

Raw apple cider vinegar. A time-honored remedy, apple cider vinegar has a variety of vitamins and minerals, and it promotes good digestion and stable blood sugar levels. You can combine it with olive oil to make a salad dressing, or add 1 tablespoon to an 8-ounce glass of water and just drink it.

Sea vegetables. Rich in minerals, including iodine, iron, and magnesium, sea vegetables may also protect against cancer (Yang et al. 2010). Try adding dulse, kombu, or kelp to soups, stews, and legume dishes. Nori, the seaweed used in sushi, is a great snack and can be used in place of tortillas to make wraps.

Miso. This fermented soybean paste has all the benefits of fermented foods and may also protect against cancer and heart disease (Murooka and Yamshita 2008). This is one of the few soy products that I recommend. And if you don't tolerate soy or need to avoid it for any reason, you can also find miso made from rice, barley, and other beans. Just make sure it's organic and raw. Don't heat miso, as this destroys its beneficial enzymes. The easiest way to get the benefits of miso is to mix 1 tablespoon into a bit of water, then add it to a bowl of soup or stew just before serving.

Summary of Quantities and Combinations to Eat Each Day

Overall, the dietary approach I recommend has you eating proteins, fats, and carbohydrates at each meal and when you're eating snacks. The amounts of protein and fat are moderate. The amount of carbohydrates is somewhat low compared to the typical Western diet.

The amount of carbohydrate is very low if you're following the third diet, so you'll need to eat more protein and fat. The recommendations on quantities of what to eat each day are simply guidelines to help you devise your own optimum antianxiety diet. Please don't get into measuring exact cups of food or counting calories. Just use the amounts to guide you, then adjust based on your experience and unique nutritional needs. Here's an example of what a well-balanced lunch or dinner plate might look like:

- One-quarter of the plate could be a piece of grilled lamb or beef or fish (protein).

- One-quarter of the plate could be a sweet potato (starchy vegetable) with melted butter (some fat), or brown rice (a grain) drizzled with olive oil (some fat).

- Half of the plate could be steamed broccoli, cauliflower, and asparagus (nonstarchy vegetables), also drizzled with butter or olive oil (more fat).

To accompany the meal, you might have a few tablespoons of sauerkraut (a bonus food) and a salad (nonstarchy vegetables and leafy greens) with mung bean sprouts (another bonus food), sliced avocado (more fat), sesame seeds (more fat), and a homemade dressing of olive oil (more fat), apple cider vinegar (another bonus food), and fresh herbs (another bonus food). This could be followed by some fresh or baked fruit, served with coconut milk or fresh cream (some fat).

Recipe and Food Resources

As you begin making changes to your diet, you may need a few new cookbooks and food-related resources to support your antianxiety approach. Here are a few that I recommend to help you get started:

- *The New Whole Foods Encyclopedia* (1999), by Rebecca Wood. This is a great resource for selection and preparation of vegetables, fruits, grains, and herbs.

- *Julia's Kitchen Wisdom* (2009), by Julia Child. This is a great little recipe book that also provides instruction in basic cooking techniques. When you're ready, also try some of her more advanced cookbooks.

- *The Bold Vegetarian: 150 Innovative International Recipes* (1995), by Bharti Kirchner. Vegetarian cookbooks can be a great resource if you're new to cooking vegetables, and this one is no exception.

- *Nourishing Traditions* (2001), by Sally Fallon. This book has recipes for many traditional meat, fish, chicken, and vegetable dishes, as well as information about and recipes for soaked, sprouted, and fermented foods, and much more.

- *Cooking to Heal: Nutrition and Cooking Class for Autism* (2010), by Julie Matthews. This recipe book and four-hour cooking DVD covers gluten-free, dairy-free, and grain-free diets, as well as traditional broths, fermented foods, and more. Julie and I have worked together, and we've found there are many overlaps between dietary approaches for autism and mental health issues, so don't be put off by the title.

With any cookbooks you use, these included, you'll need to modify the recipes to suit your own tastes and dietary needs. Here are a few specific guidelines: Replace canola and other less healthy oils with olive oil, butter, or coconut oil. Replace wheat flour with a gluten-free option. Use wheat-free tamari instead of soy sauce. Replace tofu with red meat, chicken, or fish. And, of course, just pass on any recipes that call for artificial sweeteners, processed or refined ingredients, refined sugar, or excessive amounts of natural sweeteners.

Wrapping Up

This way of eating really isn't difficult. It's more like getting back to the basics. And while any change can be hard at first, especially changes in what you eat, before you know it you'll feel great and be well on your way to eliminating anxiety. This will provide powerful motivation to stick to the diet that works for you. As a bonus, you're likely to feel enhanced overall health and well-being. Enjoy the journey of discovering the diet that works best for you.

I know this chapter has covered a lot of ground, so here are some quick reference lists to make it easier for you to design your own, personalized antianxiety food solution.

Antianxiety "Yes" Foods

- Real, whole, good-quality food, with plenty of variety

- Good-quality sources of animal protein

- Fish a few times a week

- Good fats

- Organic vegetables and fruits, in all the colors of the rainbow

- Carbohydrates from fruit, vegetables, and grains (as tolerated)

- Protein, carbohydrates, and good fats at each meal and most snacks

- Breakfast every day, with protein

- Three meals and two snacks a day

- Plenty of pure water

- Eating according to your unique biochemical needs

Antianxiety Bonus Foods

- Organ meats

- Fermented foods

- Broths

- Herbs and spices

- Other nutrient-dense foods: whey, sprouts, raw apple cider vinegar, sea vegetables, and miso

Antianxiety "Watch" Foods

- Gluten-containing grains (if tolerated), preferably soaked, sprouted, or fermented

- Dairy products (if tolerated), preferably raw and organic

- Gluten-free grains, legumes, and starchy vegetables

Antianxiety "No" Foods

- Bad fats

- Processed foods, especially those with artificial additives, preservatives, colors, and flavorings

- Coffee and other sources of caffeine

- Sugar, artificial sweeteners, and sodas

- Foods containing genetically modified ingredients

Avoid Sugar and Control Blood Sugar Swings

Eating refined sugar and other refined, processed carbohydrates and excessive fluctuations in blood sugar levels can contribute to anxiety. Addressing these factors often reduces and sometimes completely alleviates anxiety, nervousness, irritability, and feeling stressed and overwhelmed. It will also help with feeling shaky between meals or when you skip a meal.

First we'll look at refined sugar and processed foods high in sugar and why they are so harmful to your mood and your overall health. Then we'll look at blood sugar stability and how low blood sugar can mimic anxiety, which helps explain why stabilizing blood sugar levels can make such a big difference. Controlling blood sugar levels is key for the majority of my clients, anxious or not, because stable blood sugar also leads to improved overall mood, energy, mental focus and sleep, and fewer cravings.

Uncontrolled blood sugar levels can create a vicious cycle. When levels fall, you'll have increased sugar cravings, which can result in increased sugar consumption, setting you up for another spike and then drop in blood sugar level. In addition, the more sugar you eat, the more you become depleted in various nutrients, further impairing your body's ability to control blood sugar levels. This roller-coaster ride is accompanied by anxiety and mood swings. And because blood sugar swings call on the adrenal glands to produce high levels of cortisol, they ultimately stress the adrenal glands—another vicious cycle, because stressed adrenals mean worse blood sugar control. (Refer to chapter 8 for more on the adrenals.)

Sugar Consumption Questionnaire

The first step in determining whether sugar and blood sugar levels are involved in your anxiety is identifying whether you are consuming too much sugar or are addicted to sugar. This questionnaire will help you figure that out. Check off any items that apply to you. For items that mention "any other sweetener," this includes brown sugar, honey, maple syrup, date sugar, artificial sweeteners, xylitol, stevia, fructose, agave nectar, and so on (a more exhaustive list appears later in the chapter).

☐ Do you add sugar or any other sweetener to foods or beverages?

☐ Do you eat processed foods, candy, cookies, or cake containing sugar or any other sweetener?

☐ Do you drink regular sodas, diet sodas, diet drinks, sports drinks, or fruit juices?

☐ Do you enjoy something sweet after a meal or have a sweet tooth?

☐ Do you replace sugar with equal amounts of supposedly healthier sweeteners, such as honey, maple syrup, or agave nectar?

☐ Do you use xylitol, stevia, or artificial sweeteners (sucralose, aspartame, and so on)?

☐ Do you eat large quantities of fruit (ten or more servings a day)?

☐ Do you snack on dried fruit as a treat?

☐ Do you tend to overdo it with sugary foods, for example, eating a whole box of cookies rather than one or two, or a whole bar of chocolate rather than a small piece?

☐ Do you eat "white foods," such as white bread, white flour products, white pasta, and white rice, on a daily basis?

☐ Do you feel you need something sweet to feel happy, calm, comforted, or energized?

☐ Do you feel guilty about eating foods containing sugar or other sweeteners?

☐ Do you use willpower to avoid sugar and yet feel deprived?

If you checked off more than three items, you may be consuming too much sugar and other sweeteners. You may also be addicted to sugar.

The Harmful Effects of Sugar and Sweeteners

It can be hard to quit eating sugar and sweeteners. To give you more motivation, let's take a look at how sugar consumption promotes anxiety. I'll also discuss a few other health problems associated with sugar, to help you stay the course.

Blood sugar balance and anxiety. You need glucose to fuel all of your cells, especially your brain cells, but it's important to maintain relatively even blood sugar levels. Consuming refined sugar, sodas, most other sweeteners (including honey and maple syrup), and refined carbohydrates leads to a spike and then drop in blood sugar levels, which can result in anxiety, nervousness, and irritability. For now I'll leave it at that, as this topic is covered in detail later in this chapter.

Sugar, increased lactate levels, and anxiety. Sugar and alcohol may contribute to elevated levels of lactate in the blood, which can cause anxiety and panic attacks. If you suffer from anxiety, you may be more sensitive to lactate (Maddock, Carter, and Gietzen 1991). Other factors that can raise lactate levels are caffeine, food sensitivities, low levels of niacin and vitamins B_6 and B_1, or low levels of calcium and magnesium (Murray and Pizzorno 1998).

Sugar and anxiety and depression. Teens at the Appleton, Wisconsin, alternative high school were anxious, tired, angry, depressed, and difficult to manage. In 1997 nutrition and behavior expert Barbara Stitt helped implement a new school food program that included whole foods, no sugar or junk food, and water instead of sodas. Dramatic improvements were seen in mood, behavior, and school performance (Stitt 2002). Via e-mail correspondence, Barbara informed me that the healthier foods program subsequently spread to the entire school district of 15,000 students, and that one of the dramatic results was that high-school dropouts fell to just 16 per year, after averaging 450 per year previously, and all that was changed was the food. Furthermore, a study that looked at daily sugar consumption in six countries (Westover and Marangell 2002) found a strong correlation between higher consumption of sugar and increased incidence of depression. Given the link between depression and anxiety, it's possible that these results also have a bearing on anxiety.

Refined sugar and nutrient depletion. Refined sugars and sweeteners are harmful because they contain no nutrients beyond carbohydrates for energy. During refining and processing, minerals such as chromium, manganese, zinc, and magnesium are stripped away. Your body therefore has to use its own reserves of these minerals, as well as B vitamins and calcium, to digest the sugar, resulting in depletion of all of these nutrients, many of which are important for preventing anxiety and depression. Another problem is that when you fill up on sugary foods, you don't have much appetite left for nutrient-dense foods. Think about it: if you feel famished when you come home from work and eat a piece of cake, and then maybe another, do you really feel like eating dinner afterward?

Mercury toxicity and concerns about genetically modified foods. High-fructose corn syrup is a major ingredient in most processed foods, and samples of high-fructose corn syrup have been found to be tainted with mercury, a toxic metal that damages the nervous system (Dufault et al. 2009). And while we don't yet know the consequences of consuming high-fructose corn syrup and other sweeteners that are made from genetically modified corn, the safe bet is to avoid them.

Other detrimental health effects of sugar and other sweeteners. Some obvious results of overconsumption of sugar are tooth decay, diabetes, and obesity. Studies also support a link between fructose consumption and heart disease (Stanhope and Havel 2010). Sugar consumption also has an impact on immunity (Sanchez et al. 1973), attention deficit/hyperactivity disorder (Schnoll, Burshteyn, and Cea-Aravena 2003), arthritis (Darlington, Ramsey, and Mansfield 1986), and cancer (Lajous et al. 2008). In addition, in animal studies a high-glucose diet was shown to impair the production of digestive enzymes (Du, Shi, and Le 2010), and it is well-known that sugar promotes candida overgrowth (Crook 1997).

Sugars and Sweeteners Defined

It's important to understand the different types of sugars and sweeteners, their benefits, and their adverse effects, so study the following table closely. Most of the items listed affect blood sugar levels, and all can actually increase your desire for something sweet. Overconsumption of anything sweet, even fruit, isn't good for you. Even if you believe you're eating healthy sweeteners, for example, replacing refined white sugar with date sugar or honey, it's still likely that you have a problem with sugar consumption if you eat these foods often. Ideally, a moderate amount of fresh fruit should satisfy your desire for something sweet.

Sugars and Sweeteners

	Benefits	Adverse effects	Affects blood sugar?	Okay to consume?
Whole fruit	• Naturally sweet • Contains fiber • Nutrient rich	• Can be a problem with candida	Yes, if eaten alone	Great
Dried fruit	• Naturally sweet • Contains fiber • Nutrient rich	• Can be a problem with candida • Easy to eat too much	Yes, if eaten alone	In small amounts
Honey, maple syrup, molasses	• Not stripped of nutrients	• Can be a problem with candida	Yes, if eaten alone	In small amounts
Date sugar, dehydrated cane juice	• Not stripped of nutrients	• Can be a problem with candida	Yes, if eaten alone	In small amounts
Stevia	• None	• Unpleasant aftertaste	No	In small amounts
Xylitol	• Prevents tooth decay	• Can cause diarrhea	No	In small amounts
Dark chocolate	• Lowers blood pressure and lipids • Improves insulin resistance • Protects against cancer	• The sugar can be a problem with candida • Easy to eat too much • Contains caffeine	Yes, if eaten alone	In small amounts

	Benefits	Adverse effects	Affects blood sugar?	Okay to consume?
Fruit juice	• Nutrient rich	• Too high in sugar • Lacks fiber • Can be a problem with candida	Yes	Okay very diluted and not too often
Agave nectar	• None	• Raises triglycerides • Contributes to heart disease and diabetes	Yes	No
Refined sugars, processed carbohydrates	• None	• Nutrient depletion • Weight gain • Heart disease	Yes	No
High-fructose corn syrup, processed carbohydrates	• None	• Mercury toxicity • Heart disease	Yes	No
Sodas, energy drinks	• None	• Nutrient depletion • Weight gain • Heart disease	Yes	No
Artificial sweeteners	• None	• Toxicity • Weight gain	No	No

Where Sugar Is Found

Sugar is ubiquitous in processed and packaged foods. Candies, cookies, baked goods, and chocolate are obvious sources of sugar. These are interwoven into our culture: chocolate hearts and other candies on Valentine's Day, chocolate bunnies and more candy at Easter, Fourth of July treats, way too many Halloween candies, pies at Thanksgiving, and then more at Christmas. There are office and school treats on birthdays and at going-away parties. You may also treat yourself to cookies, doughnuts, ice cream, or other sweet treats for no reason at all, or maybe to help you feel better. You may treat your loved ones to something sweet, and they may treat you.

Sodas and other sugar-sweetened drinks are the number one source of added sugars in the American diet (Johnson et al. 2009). The Harvard School of Public Health, Department of Nutrition (2009) has a guide you can download that will show you just how much sugar there is, added or naturally occurring, in sodas, sports drinks, and other store-bought beverages, including fruit juices. Some of the worst offenders have over 50 grams of sugar in a 12-ounce serving, which is equivalent to about 10 teaspoons—almost ¼ cup of sugar. Even 100 percent fruit juices can have very high amounts of sugar, so it isn't a good idea to consume them regularly. If you do drink fruit juice, diluting it with water is a good idea, using just one part juice to eight parts water. If you avoid all of these beverages, you'll reduce your sugar consumption drastically. Instead, try healthy alternatives like iced filtered water with a splash of lemon or lime juice or unsweetened cranberry juice; filtered water with slices of orange or a few mashed strawberries; herbal teas like mint, ginger, or licorice, either hot or iced; green tea; fermented drinks like kombucha and water kefir (which is dairy-free); and coffee substitutes.

Perhaps less obvious, but very widespread, is the addition of sugar and other sweeteners to processed foods. I encourage you to look at items in your pantry: ketchup, salad dressings, peanut butter, packaged meals, instant soups, and even products with meat in them. If you eat processed foods or eat out, you're consuming added sugar, usually in the form of high-fructose corn syrup. If, on the other hand, you eat real, whole foods, you won't be getting all of those added sugars and sweeteners.

If you do buy packaged or processed foods, read labels carefully. You can equate any of the following ingredients with just plain sugar. If any of them are among the first five items in the ingredients list, that food is almost assuredly high in sugar:

- agave nectar
- barley malt
- brown sugar
- corn syrup
- dehydrated cane juice
- dextrin
- dextrose
- fructose
- fruit juice concentrate
- glucose
- high-fructose corn syrup
- honey
- invert sugar
- isomalt
- lactose
- maltodextrin
- maltose
- malt syrup
- maple syrup
- molasses
- raw sugar
- rice syrup
- saccharose
- sucrose
- syrup
- turbinado sugar
- xylose

Packaged foods may contain what you'd consider "healthy" sugars, such as fruit juice, maple syrup, or honey, but they are still sugars, and when digested they affect blood sugar in the same way. Agave nectar is used extensively as a "healthy" alternative to sugar these days. I don't recommend it. It's highly processed and also consists primarily of fructose, so it has the potential to raise triglycerides and contribute to heart disease and diabetes (Stanhope and Havel 2010).

Refined grains, such as white flour and white rice, are also problematic. Because they lack fiber, they're digested faster than other complex carbohydrates. Their sugars are released into the bloodstream more rapidly, so they affect blood sugar in much the same way as sugar. They are also lower in nutrients such as vitamin E and the B vitamins. Refined grains show up in many places—not just white bread, but also pasta, many flour tortillas, and even in many breads labeled "whole wheat."

Artificial Sweeteners

Don't replace sugar with artificial sweeteners, such as acesulfame K, aspartame, neotame, saccharin, and sucralose. They can actually contribute to weight gain because they increase appetite, and because they are sweet they also encourage sugar cravings (Yang 2010). And because they aren't real foods, some people are sensitive to them and experience adverse reactions. For example, aspartame causes headaches, insomnia, dizziness, general feelings of malaise, and, for those with mood disorders, worsening depression and nervousness (Bradstock et al. 1986; Humphries, Pretorius, and Naudé 2008). For more information on the harmful effects of artificial sweeteners, as well as MSG and other food additives, check out *Excitotoxins: The Taste that Kills* (1997), by Russell Blaylock.

What to Use Instead of Unhealthy Sugars and Artificial Sweeteners

In place of sugar and artificially sweetened foods, enjoy healthy organic fruit and sweet starchy vegetables like sweet potatoes. Coconut has a pleasing flavor that's naturally almost sweet. Spices like cinnamon and licorice can also help satisfy a sweet tooth. In terms of added sweeteners, the only options I'd consider remotely healthy are raw honey, maple syrup, molasses, homemade applesauce, or freshly squeezed fruit juice, and even these should only be consumed only in very small quantities, not as one-for-one substitutions for sugar, as they do affect blood sugar. Also, be aware that some honey is made by bees who are fed sugar; research any honey you buy and avoid this type. And although dried fruit may seem like a good option, it has a high sugar content, and it's easy to eat too much.

In 2009, the American Heart Association released a statement on the ill effects of sugar and some guidelines for consumption (Johnson et al. 2009). They suggest an upper limit of 6 teaspoons of added sugars per day for women and 9 teaspoons per day for men. While this is a major improvement on the current average of 22 teaspoons a day, my recommendation is to avoid any added sugar or limit your consumption to 2 or 3 teaspoons at most, in the form of honey, maple syrup, or molasses.

There are two sweeteners that don't affect blood sugar: xylitol (a sugar alcohol) and stevia (an herb). However, I still recommend that you use them sparingly, if at all. Because they are sweet, both promote a sweet tooth and encourage sugar cravings. Another downside is that sugar alcohols can cause diarrhea.

Dark chocolate needs a special mention because chocolate is so popular—and so highly touted for its health benefits these days. Chocolate does improve mood and create feelings of joy (Macht and Dettmer 2006). And dark chocolate does have health benefits. Moderate consumption has been shown to lower blood pressure, decrease levels of lipids in the blood, have anti-inflammatory properties, and improve insulin resistance (a condition characterized by decreased sensitivity to insulin and associated with diabetes), all of which could be beneficial for heart health (Corti et al. 2010). Dark chocolate may also offer protection against cancer (Maskarinec 2009). But the big question is, can you eat just one piece? If not, you need to figure out why. If you overindulge to comfort or calm yourself or to improve your mood, use the information on brain chemistry in chapter 6 to find out why. Also, chocolate contains caffeine and may cause migraines. Dark chocolate that is at least 70 percent cocoa is the best choice because it has less sugar and more cocoa, which is rich in antioxidants and flavonols (a class of plant-based compounds that provide many of the same benefits as antioxidants).

If you want to control your anxiety, it's critical that you avoid sugar altogether. This means not adding sugar to anything, or using it only sparingly. It means no cake, candy, or sweet foods, no sugary drinks, no processed foods, and no artificial sweeteners. Instead, eat real food, and eat to control your blood sugar. (I'll explain how to do that in the next section.)

Ideally, you shouldn't have a sweet tooth, and you should not be seeking out the next "healthy" sweetener that comes on the market. If you do, it's a message that you need to address your diet, nutrient deficiencies, imbalanced brain chemistry or even an addiction (see chapter 6), or candida (see chapter 5). This applies whether you're craving "healthy" sweeteners, sugar, or something with artificial sweeteners.

Control Blood Sugar Swings

In his book *Nutrition and Mental Illness* (1987), physician and biochemist Carl Pfeiffer emphasized that blood sugar balance is crucial. You need to provide your brain with glucose so it can function. When it doesn't get the glucose it needs, you can suffer from the many emotional and physical signs of low blood sugar (hypoglycemia), including anxiety and depression (Harp and Fox 1990).

Low Blood Sugar Questionnaire

This questionnaire will help you identify whether you may be suffering from low blood sugar. Check off any of the following symptoms that you experience on a daily basis:

☐ Nervousness or anxiety

☐ Feeling stressed and overwhelmed

☐ Phobias and fears

☐ Irritability or agitation

☐ Depression or mood swings

☐ Feeling shaky between meals or when you skip a meal

☐ Poor memory and concentration

☐ Fatigue

☐ Generally feeling better after eating

☐ Intense cravings for sweets

☐ Cravings for carbohydrates or alcohol

☐ Needing coffee to get going in the morning or to keep your energy up

☐ Insomnia or waking during the night

If you checked off more than three items, it's possible that you may be suffering from low blood sugar. If these symptoms often appear three to five hours after eating, it's especially likely that they're due to low blood sugar. This questionnaire is based on my experience working with many clients, along with information from *Nutrition and Mental Illness* (1987), by Carl Pfeiffer; and *Textbook of Natural Medicine* (2000), by Joseph Pizzorno and Michael Murray.

Benefits of Controlling Blood Sugar Swings

When you have stable blood sugar, you'll feel grounded, experience less anxiety, and feel less overwhelmed and stressed. There's also a good chance that you'll have fewer or no sugar cravings, though they may still occur if they're due to other brain chemistry imbalances (see chapter 6) or candida (see chapter 5), rather than blood sugar fluctuations.

Low blood sugar is a controversial topic, and there isn't universal agreement about how low blood sugar can fall before being considered abnormal. There are even questions about whether symptoms such as those in the previous questionnaire are caused by swings in blood sugar. So don't be surprised if your doctor isn't convinced that your anxiety may be related to low blood sugar. However, holistic health practitioners do recognize the connection and always include stabilizing blood sugar levels in their approach to healing. In fact, in *Anxiety: Orthomolecular Diagnosis and Treatment* (2006), Jonathan Prousky, a naturopath and specialist in neurological health, has written about the importance of evaluating for this if you have anxiety.

As many as twenty million Americans may suffer from low blood sugar, or hypoglycemia. *Reactive hypoglycemia* is the most common form; it typically occurs three to five hours after eating sugar or high-carbohydrate foods (Pizzorno and Murray 2000). Alcohol can also be involved in hypoglycemia. Many alcoholics are more prone to abnormal swings in blood sugar, resulting in anxiety, shakiness, fatigue, and increased cravings for alcohol or sugar (Ketcham and Mueller 1983).

Simple Dietary Changes to Help Control Blood Sugar Swings

If the previous questionnaire indicates low blood sugar may be an issue for you, try the dietary approaches outlined next. They're simple enough, and you may be surprised at how much better you feel after implementing them. I also encourage you to keep a food log (see appendix 2 for a form you can use). By writing down what you eat and when you eat, and monitoring how you feel afterward, you'll develop a better understanding of your situation. If you notice that you tend to feel shaky and anxious after not eating for a while, you may need to eat more frequently. Initially, you may even need to eat every two or three hours.

Avoid sugar, processed foods, and "white foods." It should go without saying: Avoid junk food, refined sugar, all of the white foods (white flour, white rice, white bread, and so on), processed foods, sodas, sugary beverages, and alcohol. Following the recommendations earlier in this chapter and in chapter 1 is the first step in stabilizing blood sugar. Focus on real, whole foods, choose unrefined complex carbohydrates (such as brown rice), and make sure to include high-fiber foods (such as legumes and vegetables) in your diet.

Eat enough protein. One of the most important things I tell all of my anxious clients is to eat enough protein. We all have unique needs, but a good rule of thumb for blood sugar control and optimal mental health is to eat at least 3 to 4 ounces of quality protein at each meal; that's the amount in a palm-size portion. For more details, see the guidelines for protein consumption in chapter 1.

Eat breakfast, and have protein at breakfast. The next important thing is to eat breakfast every day, within an hour of waking, being sure to include protein, such as eggs, fish, chicken sausage, or yogurt. Avoid processed, packaged cereals; instead, eat real oatmeal, buckwheat, or any other whole grains you tolerate well, with nuts, seeds, coconut, butter, or kefir, or a scoop of whey or rice protein powder for more rounded nutrition. Smoothies can be a good breakfast too, especially if you don't have a big appetite in the morning.

A good recipe includes filtered water as the base, ¼ cup of full-fat coconut milk, fruit (such as organic raspberries or blueberries), and at least 20 grams of whey or rice protein powder. Simply blend and enjoy. Some other optional ingredients for your smoothie are freshly juiced greens or a greens powder, yogurt or kefir, nut butter, and freshly ground flaxseeds. If you drink coffee, make sure to eat breakfast first, or the coffee will reduce your appetite. (However, I encourage you to avoid caffeine, as discussed in chapter 3.)

Eat at least three meals and two snacks daily. Eat at least three good-quality meals and two good-quality snacks daily, making sure to include protein, fat, and carbohydrate in each meal and most snacks to help keep blood sugar levels stable. Just to review, meat, poultry, eggs, and dairy products are good sources of protein; butter, olive oil, avocado, and coconut provide healthy fats; and brown rice or starchy vegetables like sweet potatoes or carrots provide carbohydrates, as do fruits. From these basic building blocks, you can assemble a wide variety of meals: roasted chicken with the skin (a source of fat) and vegetables; a big salad with leafy greens, vegetables, avocado, and fish; or a beef stew with lots of vegetables, served on brown rice and drizzled with olive oil. Here are some great snack ideas: a boiled egg, whole grain or rice crackers and hummus, grass-fed jerky, pemmican, fruit and a few nuts, whole-grain crackers and cheese, and raw carrots or zucchini with cream cheese. If you're prone to low blood sugar, always carry some nuts with you for emergency snacks.

Have a bedtime snack. If you wake up anxious and hungry at night, you may have a problem with nighttime low blood sugar. Eating a light snack just before bed can be helpful. Try different food combinations to find what works best for you. Try half a banana (bananas contain tryptophan, which promotes sleep), alone or with 1 tablespoon of nut butter, such as almond butter or tahini. Other good bedtime snacks would be a small piece of cheese or a slice of fruit, such as apple—or try cheese and fruit together. Although sleep problems can have many causes other than low blood sugar, a bedtime snack is worth trying, and it just might help you sleep through the night. Other causes of nighttime waking are high cortisol (covered in the section on the adrenals in chapter 8), food sensitivities (see chapter 4), caffeine (see chapter 3), low serotonin or low GABA (see chapter 6), or digestive problems (see chapter 5).

Supplements

If dietary changes aren't enough to control your blood sugar, there are two supplements that can help: the mineral chromium and the amino acid glutamine.

Chromium. Because chromium plays a fundamental role in controlling blood sugar levels, it can help relieve symptoms of reactive hypoglycemia (Anderson et al. 1987). It works by increasing the action of insulin, the hormone that controls transfer of glucose from the bloodstream into the cells, where it can be used for energy. This also helps explain why chromium is depleted by a high-sugar diet. Chromium also helps raise levels of the neurotransmitter serotonin and has been shown to alleviate atypical depression, a form of depression that includes an increase in appetite and weight gain (Davidson et al. 2003). Chromium could, therefore, also improve anxiety that is related to low levels of serotonin. Make sure your multivitamin contains at least 200 mcg (micrograms) of chromium. If you have severe blood sugar swings, you can take additional chromium to help stabilize levels; an extra 200 mcg of chromium with meals often helps.

Glutamine. The amino acid glutamine provides fuel or energy for your brain when your blood sugar dips too low, and reduces cravings for sugar, carbohydrates, and alcohol and improve glucose metabolism (Braverman 2003). Try taking 500 to 1,500 mg (milligrams) two or three times a day, between meals. (But first, please review the general precautions about supplementing with amino acids in chapter 6.) For a quick effect, open the capsules, put the powder on your tongue, and allow it to dissolve (Ross 2004). I have found this to be very effective for many of my clients. Glutamine is also very healing for the digestive system (Miller 1999), so it will provide additional benefits if you have digestive issues (see chapter 5) or damage to your digestive system from food sensitivities (see chapter 4). Avoid glutamine if you have bipolar disorder, as it may trigger an episode of mania (Mebane 1984).

■ Theresa's Story

Theresa described her sugar cravings as an "almost demonic urge to eat sugar and all things sweet." Making changes to her diet and trying to control her blood sugar levels by eating the right foods at the right times wasn't enough to eliminate her cravings. However, she did find that taking glutamine whenever she felt the urge to eat something sweet made a difference. Opening a 500 mg capsule onto her tongue was more effective than swallowing the capsule. We had the same conversation that I have with all clients who would obviously rather eat something sweet than open a glutamine capsule onto their tongues. I told her, "If you have a craving, tell yourself that you're going to indulge, but also humor your nutritionist and take the glutamine anyway. You may be surprised to find your urge completely disappears." Theresa was pleasantly surprised to find that it worked for her. She recently wrote me to report on a few other changes that had been pivotal to her recovery: "...exercise, improved sleep, meditation, and affirmations. Add to that a personal tenacity, an unwillingness to give up, and a deep desire to conquer this lifelong foe."

How Quickly You Can Expect Improvements

For many of my clients, changing to a wholesome diet as described in chapter 1, making the changes described in this chapter, and eliminating caffeine (discussed in chapter 3) is enough for them to experience a complete turnaround in anxiety, often in a week or less. In addition, they often experience increased energy, reduced cravings, better sleep, and improved overall health and well-being.

If You Have a Sugar or Carb Addiction and Can't Quit

If you've tried all the recommendations in this chapter and still can't give up sugar, you may be addicted. Sugar, as well as refined foods and fatty foods, can truly be as addicting as substances like alcohol and tobacco (Ifland et al. 2009), and these kinds of food addictions are often associated with an increased risk for depression, anxiety, weight gain, and substance abuse (Corwin and Grigson 2009).

If you have an addiction to sugar and other sweeteners and can't stop consuming them, despite the fact that you know that this is unhealthy and perhaps don't feel so great after indulging, it doesn't mean you're a failure, a weak person, or lacking in willpower. If staying away from sugar makes you feel deprived, you feel driven to eat sugar, or you yo-yo between eating well and then indulging, addressing the underlying causes can end your sugar cravings and addiction.

One solution may be to balance your brain chemistry; chapter 6 will help you assess whether you have a neurotransmitter imbalance and are perhaps using sugar to alter your mood or physiology. (Using any substance in this way is often referred to as *self-medicating*.) For example, you may have low levels of GABA (leading you to eat sugar to relieve stress and anxiety), low serotonin (resulting in afternoon and evening cravings and leading you to eat sugar to improve your mood), low catecholamines (making you eat sugar for energy), or low endorphins (inclining you to eat to comfort yourself). When you correct these imbalances, your cravings will diminish and eventually disappear, along with mood problems related to deficient neurotransmitters, including anxiety. *The Diet Cure* (2011) is a great resource for neurotransmitter imbalances and cravings.

Another solution may be to address candida and dysbiosis (discussed in chapter 5). Both can cause intense sugar cravings because both candida and "unfriendly" intestinal bacteria feed on sugar. If your cravings revolve around cookies, cake, or bread, gluten sensitivity may be an issue you need to address (discussed in chapter 4). Also look at the section on adrenal health in chapter 8, as blood sugar control and adrenal function are closely interrelated.

CHAPTER 3

Avoid Caffeine, Alcohol, and Nicotine

Some people are more sensitive to caffeine and experience adverse reactions, including increased anxiety, nervousness, and sleep problems. And even if caffeine doesn't make you feel anxious, I encourage you to consider its other ill effects and refrain from using it. There are also links between alcohol and nicotine use and anxiety. Because these substances alter both mood and physiology, people tend to turn to them to help change how they're feeling (as discussed in chapter 2, this is self-medication). But all three have significant downsides and usually end up doing more harm than good, in terms of anxiety, and overall health and well-being. All three—caffeine, alcohol, and nicotine—are mood-altering drugs that damage the brain (Hyman 2009). If you use caffeine, alcohol, or nicotine, I encourage you to work through this chapter to make a change.

Coffee and Caffeine

In 2009, the National Coffee Association reported that just over 50 percent of U.S. adults drink coffee. Worldwide, coffee is one of the most consumed beverages, and high-caffeine energy drinks (which are also loaded with sugar) are becoming increasingly popular.

Although it's legal, caffeine is really a stimulant drug. It elevates heart rate, increases blood flow, raises body temperature and blood sugar, and acts as a diuretic, and people often experience withdrawal symptoms when they stop using caffeine. It's often used for self-medication, with people altering how much they use based on their needs. And as with most other drugs, with time you build up tolerance, so you'll need more and more to produce the same energizing effect.

The double whammy of caffeine and sugar in energy drinks and sweetened coffee has an even bigger impact on the body. Other ingredients added to coffee are also problematic; for example, synthetic coffee creamers are full of processed nonfoods. Soy milk has become a popular replacement for milk in lattes and the like, yet soy has its own set of problems, discussed in chapter 1. Beyond coffee and energy drinks, caffeine is also found in black tea, many sodas, yerba maté tea, guarana, certain medications (weight-loss aids and pain medications, like Excedrin), and, in smaller amounts, in green and white tea. Even decaf coffee contains a small amount of caffeine. Caffeine is also found in all forms of chocolate and cacao (other than white chocolate); the darker the chocolate, the more caffeine it contains.

Caffeine and Anxiety

Many people have experienced that caffeine consumption can worsen anxiety, and there's solid scientific evidence to support this link. For example, chronic, heavy use of caffeine can cause or heighten anxiety and may lead to increased use of antianxiety medications (Clementz and Dailey 1988). Like sugar, caffeine can lead to higher levels of lactate in your blood. If you're sensitive to lactate buildup, it may make you more prone to anxiety and panic attacks (Pizzorno and Murray 2000). People with panic disorder and social anxiety may be more sensitive to the anxiety-causing effects of caffeine (Lara 2010).

The side effects of excessive caffeine intake are numerous and well documented: increased heart rate, restlessness, anxiety, depression, tremors, difficulty sleeping, excessive urination, and nausea (MedlinePlus 2009). Excessive intake is defined as ten 8-ounce cups of coffee a day, which I've found to be quite common. But for some people, much less than this—even just a few sips—can have similar effects (Clementz and Dailey 1988). And, somewhat paradoxically, caffeine withdrawal can also mimic anxiety (Greden 1974). Many people experience withdrawal when they stop using caffeine (Juliano and Griffiths 2004). Symptoms may include headache, fatigue, decreased energy and focus, drowsiness, depressed mood, irritability, and even flu-like symptoms, nausea, and muscle stiffness.

In a study comparing people with panic disorders and agoraphobia to healthy subjects, those with panic disorders experienced increases in symptoms such as nervousness, fear, nausea, heart palpitations, and tremors after consuming caffeine and said the effects were similar to how they felt during a panic attack (Charney, Heninger, and Jatlow 1985). The control group didn't experience these effects. Another study (Bruce and Lader 1989) looked at four men and two women with generalized anxiety and panic disorder, none of whom had benefited from drug therapy or psychotherapy. All consumed caffeine—from 1½ to 3½ cups of coffee a day. They stopped drinking coffee, and within a week their anxiety disappeared. I've seen similar results in many of my clients. Sometimes this is the only change that anxious people need to make. It's certainly worth a try.

Other Reasons to Consider Giving Up Caffeine

Coffee proponents are fond of citing studies showing that caffeine increases energy, elevates mood, and may improve cognition, reduce stroke risk, and even delay Alzheimer's disease. Still, I encourage you to just eat more oily fish, such as salmon, and plenty of vegetables and fruits. You'll get all the same benefits without the following side effects.

- Caffeine can disrupt sleep, especially when you indulge within a few hours of bedtime, because of its stimulating effects and because it depletes serotonin and melatonin (Ross 2002), both of which promote restful sleep. As a result, you're more likely to need caffeine to keep you going the next day. And because caffeine is a diuretic, you'll probably have an increased need to urinate during the night, which may also affect your sleep.

- Caffeine can aggravate the symptoms of PMS (Clementz and Dailey 1988) and cause increased breast tenderness.

- Caffeine depletes the B vitamins, vitamin C, potassium, magnesium, calcium, and zinc.

- Caffeine causes the adrenal glands to produce more epinephrine and norepinephrine, and over time, this will weaken the adrenals (Levi 1967).

- In animal studies, caffeine has been shown to elevate levels of testosterone and estradiol (Celec and Behuliak 2010), which could create hormone imbalances.

How to Quit Caffeine and What to Drink Instead

I have many clients who are very health conscious and wouldn't dream of drinking sodas but find it difficult to even consider giving up coffee. Many are initially reluctant to give it up, since it usually gives them an energy boost and they enjoy the taste, the aroma, and their coffee-making rituals. However, this usually changes once they quit and find they have less anxiety, or no anxiety at all.

If you find yourself similarly reluctant to give up caffeine, you need to address why you need it as a pick-me-up. You may have underlying tiredness for a variety of reasons: food sensitivities (chapter 4), low catecholamines (chapter 6), adrenal fatigue, an underactive thyroid, anemia, or simply not getting enough sleep (all covered in chapter 8). If you can't function without your morning coffee or need caffeine to be productive through the day, it's important to get to the root cause of your fatigue.

Be forewarned: quitting can be tough, but I do have a few suggestions for how you can make it easier. When you're quitting, take extra vitamin C (at least 1,000 mg three times a day). If you have signs of low catecholamines, such as depression with lethargy, low energy, poor focus, low motivation, and cravings for sugar and caffeine for energy, take 500 to 1,500 mg of tyrosine three times daily: first thing in the morning, midmorning, and midafternoon. If you decide to take tyrosine, please refer to the general precautions about supplementing with amino acids in chapter 6.

You can either quit cold turkey and stop caffeine all at once or gradually reduce your consumption over about a week. It's good to have some alternative beverages on hand. Instead of coffee or black tea, try delicious herbal teas (such as licorice, lemon-ginger, and mint), coffee substitutes such as Dandy Blend, magnesium-rich carob, and green rooibos (an herbal tea from South Africa that appears to have health benefits similar to those of green tea). Instead of sodas, drink filtered water, fermented beverages like kombucha, and herbal iced teas.

If You Do Want to Drink Coffee

If caffeine doesn't make you anxious or affect your sleep and you don't suffer from adrenal fatigue, you may decide you still want to drink coffee despite its other side effects. If so, it's still a good idea to be moderate and drink it only occasionally. Also, make sure you drink organic coffee, as conventionally grown coffee is heavily sprayed with pesticides. Another option is to purchase shade-grown coffee; this is the traditional way of growing coffee and often requires fewer pesticides. If you choose to drink decaffeinated coffee, be aware that small amounts of caffeine do remain. Also, select water process decaffeinated, rather than solvent processed, which uses potentially toxic chemicals. If you have coffee in the morning, drink it after you've eaten breakfast so it doesn't reduce your appetite. And do consider green tea as a healthier alternative to coffee.

■ Dee's Story

When Dee first came to see me, she was anxious, depressed, and very tired, and she suffered from PMS. She was drinking eight to ten cups of coffee a day, just so she could get through her day. We identified and addressed some of the main reasons for her fatigue: poor blood sugar control, which she remedied by eating healthy snacks, and anemia, for which she started taking iron supplements. She also supplemented with amino acids (see chapter 6): GABA for the anxiety, tyrosine for low energy, and 5-hydroxytryptophan (5-HTP) for her low mood. She started to feel much better within a few weeks and was able to function without coffee—so much so that a few weeks later she spent two days spring-cleaning her home!

Getting to the root cause of her fatigue allowed Dee to function very well without coffee. When she quit, she did experience some reduction in anxiety, but she also benefited from the calming effects of supplemental GABA and 5-HTP. In addition, she felt more optimistic, was sleeping better, and had fewer sugar cravings. Later, when she decided to try the occasional cup of coffee, she discovered that it made her feel very anxious. That made it easier for her to stay away from it.

Alcohol

Alcohol has been shown to contribute to increased feelings of anxiety (Monteiro, Schuckit, and Irwin 1990), so if you already suffer from anxiety, you should avoid it. Alcohol also causes nutritional deficiencies, often results in reactive hypoglycemia, and can cause reactions similar to food sensitivities—all of which can make your anxiety worse. In addition, if you have pyroluria (discussed in chapter 7), low histamine (discussed in chapter 4), or a family history of alcoholism, it's likely that you'll have difficulty tolerating alcohol.

Nutritional Deficiencies Due to Alcohol Consumption

Alcohol can cause nutritional deficiencies for two reasons: the effects of alcohol in the body and skipped meals while drinking. Many of the nutrients it depletes are important for preventing anxiety (Pizzorno and Murray 2000): zinc, vitamin C, magnesium, fatty acids, antioxidants, and the stress-busting B vitamins, such as B_6 (pyridoxine), B_1 (thiamine), and folic acid. Alcohol consumption adversely affects the metabolism of tryptophan (the precursor for serotonin), leading to lowered levels of serotonin, an important neurotransmitter. This has been linked to anger and even violence (Badawy 2003), and may also contribute to anxiety, depression, sleep problems, and cravings.

Alcohol and Low Blood Sugar

Alcohol causes reactive hypoglycemia—a drop in blood sugar shortly after and up to twelve hours after consumption—which will leave you craving sugar or more alcohol. However, sugar and alcohol consumption will only aggravate the situation, leading to symptoms of low blood sugar, such as anxiety, dizziness, headache, and fatigue. (See chapter 2 for more on low blood sugar.)

Alcohol Sensitivity

You may react to certain ingredients, such as sulfites in wine, or wheat, rye, barley, or corn in beer and distilled liquors (Vally and Thompson 2003). Typical reactions involve respiratory symptoms like asthma, sneezing, headaches, and itching. In addition, these reactions can affect your sleep, potentially leading to anxiety, depression, and alcohol abuse (Nathan 2007). You can use the food sensitivity information in chapter 4 to help determine your particular issue and what to do.

How to Quit Alcohol

The approach to quitting drinking is the same as for any addiction. The key is balancing your brain chemistry. Amino acids can be very helpful. This is the topic of chapter 6, so I won't give full details here. But here's a quick overview: The amino acid glutamine is particularly helpful for quitting alcohol because it reduces the desire to drink and also helps stabilize blood sugar. Plus, glutamine is very healing for the gut, which pays a heavy toll when you consume alcohol. If you drink to improve your mood, supplementing with tryptophan or 5-HTP may help. If you drink for energy, tyrosine may help. And if you drink to calm down, GABA may help. Supplementing with the amino acid taurine can also be helpful, as it prevents alcohol withdrawal symptoms and reduces alcohol damage to the liver (Braverman 2003). Taurine is often low in people with depression, and because it's also calming, it will also help with anxiety, which often coexists with depression and addictions.

Nicotine

The harmful effects of smoking are well publicized and well known. In brief, it increases the body's load of those damaging, reactive molecules known as free radicals and causes cancer, emphysema, and heart disease. It also increases heart rate and blood pressure. Some smokers experience increased irritability and poor concentration. Smoking and exposure to secondhand smoke deplete vitamin C, vitamin E, folic acid, and vitamin B_1. And because smoking also reduces your appetite and affects your taste perception, it often results in further nutritional deficiencies.

Nicotine and Anxiety

A study looking at adolescent smokers (Goodwin, Lewinsohn, and Seeley 2005) found that they had an increased risk of panic attacks and panic disorder in early adulthood. Although smoking may temporarily relieve anxiety, in the long run it results in increased nervousness and agitation, which often resolve upon quitting. In one study (West and Hajek 1997), there was a significant decrease in anxiety after the first week of abstinence.

How to Quit Smoking

As with drinking, the key to quitting smoking is to balance your brain chemistry. Refer to chapter 6 for all the information on how to use amino acids to help you quit. Doing this in conjunction with hypnotherapy or guided imagery (Wynd 2005) is often the most effective approach.

How Quickly You Can Expect Improvements

Abstaining from caffeine, alcohol, and nicotine can help alleviate anxiety, and also improve your sleep and overall mood, often within a week. If you balance your brain chemistry and address nutrient deficiencies, you won't end up replacing one craving (for caffeine, alcohol, or nicotine) with another (for sugar or carbohydrates, for example).

CHAPTER 4

Address Problems with Gluten and Other Food Sensitivities

Food sensitivities can have effects beyond physiological symptoms, including creating imbalances in key chemicals in the brain (Pfeiffer 1987), which can cause anxiety, phobias, depression, irritability, and mood swings. When food sensitivities have these effects, they are sometimes termed "brain allergies" or "cerebral allergies" (ibid; Rippere 1984).

While substances such as sugar, caffeine, and alcohol are highly likely to affect mood and behavior, food sensitivities appear to have these sorts of effects on certain susceptible individuals, causing increased anxiety and other psychological symptoms, as well as increased heart rate (King 1984). This chapter will help you determine if that might be the case for you. You'll often find the terms "food sensitivity" and "food intolerance" used interchangeably. For simplicity's sake, I'll use the term "food sensitivity" in this chapter.

Food Sensitivities Questionnaire

This questionnaire will help you identify whether food sensitivities could be contributing to your anxiety or causing other emotional or physiological symptoms, including digestive problems. Check off any of the following signs and symptoms that apply to you on a regular basis:

Part 1: Signs and Symptoms

☐ Anxiety, fear, panic attacks, or social phobia

☐ Depression

☐ Excessive daily mood swings or bipolar disorder

☐ Preferring to eat certain foods daily, such as bread, pasta, cheese, or ice cream

☐ Fatigue or drowsiness, especially after eating

☐ Asthma, congestion, postnasal drip, or hay fever

☐ Sensitivity to food dyes and additives, showing up in symptoms such as rashes or headaches

☐ Insomnia

☐ Digestive problems like gas, bloating, constipation, or diarrhea

☐ Migraines or chronic headaches

☐ Rashes, eczema, dermatitis, or psoriasis

☐ Frequent colds and infections

Part 2: Conditions

☐ Iron-deficiency anemia or low ferritin

☐ Other nutrient deficiencies, particularly low vitamin D

☐ Inability to gain weight

☐ History of colic as a child

☐ Celiac disease, wheat or gluten sensitivity, or known issues with eating wheat or dairy

☐ Having first-degree family members (mother, father, sister, brother, son, or daughter) with celiac disease or gluten sensitivity

☐ Type 1 diabetes or autoimmune thyroiditis

☐ Having first-degree family members with type 1 diabetes or autoimmune thyroiditis

☐ High whole blood histamine or seasonal environmental allergies

☐ Low whole blood histamine or known food sensitivities

☐ Pyroluria (see chapter 7)

☐ Osteopenia, osteoporosis, or frequent bone fractures

☐ Infertility, history of miscarriage, or having a baby with low birth weight

☐ Epilepsy

☐ Fibromyalgia or a neuromuscular condition, such as ataxia

☐ Autism spectrum disorder or learning disorder, including attention deficit disorder or attention deficit/hyperactivity disorder

☐ Schizophrenia or abnormal thinking

If you checked off five or more items in each section, I encourage you to use this chapter to determine whether food sensitivities may be a factor in your anxiety. It may be worthwhile to be tested for celiac disease too. At a minimum, do the elimination-challenge trials as described, or find a nutritionist who can guide you through the process.

This questionnaire is based on my clinical experience working with clients with mood problems, food sensitivities, and celiac disease, along with information from *Nutrition and Mental Illness* (1987), by Carl

Pfeiffer; *Digestive Wellness* (2004), by Elizabeth Lipski; and *Dangerous Grains* (2002), by James Braly and Ron Hoggan.

Why Food May Be Affecting Your Mood

Problem foods can contribute to anxiety in a number of ways, including inflammation and physical stress due to the production of antibodies. Another possible mechanism relates to histamine, a compound involved in the immune response and that also functions as a neurotransmitter. A histamine imbalance is often related to allergies or sensitivities to both foods and environmental allergens, such as pollen, dander, or mold (Pfeiffer 1987; Jackson et al. 1998).

Gluten sensitivity can limit the availability of tryptophan and therefore lead to decreases in levels of serotonin (Pynnönen et al. 2005). (See chapter 6 for more on the link between serotonin and anxiety.) Another possible mechanism is indirect effects of gastrointestinal damage due to eating problem foods, resulting in nutrient malabsorption (Hallert et al. 2009). And yet another is an effect wherein you're drawn to eat certain foods to get a psychological high (Pfeiffer 1987) caused by gluteomorphins—opiate-like compounds produced during the digestion of the gliadin component of the gluten protein. Gluteomorphins are addicting, and withdrawal symptoms can feel as bad as drug withdrawal. When you consume gluten, initially you'll feel great, but then you'll experience a severe letdown that may show up as anxiety, depression, mood swings, fatigue, and other symptoms.

In my work with anxious clients, the foods that most often seem to be involved in anxiety and other mood problems are those that contain gluten. Gluten is found primarily in wheat, rye, and barley, and oats may be contaminated with gluten during processing and transportation. Less commonly, people may have difficulty with a wide range of carbohydrates, including all grains and starchy vegetables. Although dairy doesn't directly contribute to mood problems, people with gluten issues often also have trouble with dairy because of damage to the digestive system. In this chapter I'll primarily cover gluten and only touch on dairy and other food issues. But remember, because each of us is biochemically unique, almost any food could be an issue for you—physically, emotionally, or both. I'll explain how you can identify which foods you may be sensitive to.

If you discover that you have sensitivities to certain foods, it's best to avoid those foods for at least three months. Then you can slowly reincorporate them into your diet one by one and monitor how you feel after adding each one. Some foods may always be a problem for you, but you could find that you can eat others on a rotational basis, perhaps once every two or three days. Be aware that it's possible to develop sensitivities to foods that you eat day in and day out. So aim for variety and rotate the foods you eat, especially those you've been sensitive to.

Celiac disease (a subset of gluten sensitivity) is an autoimmune disorder caused by a reaction to gluten and merits a special note. If you test positive for celiac disease, you'll need to avoid gluten for life; this is currently the only treatment known to be effective. Celiac disease is associated with many serious health problems, including rheumatoid arthritis, fibromyalgia, dermatitis herpetiformis, eczema, epilepsy, colon cancer, and thyroid abnormalities (Braly and Hoggan 2002). Also, those with untreated celiac disease have been found to have reduced blood flow to certain areas of the brain (Addolorato et al. 2004). This could have a bearing on anxiety, depression, and cognitive functions, such as focus. If you have celiac disease and continue to eat gluten, it will probably affect your quality of life and may shorten your life (Corrao et al. 2001). Even if you don't have a diagnosis of celiac disease, if you feel better when you don't eat gluten, I recommend avoiding it to prevent possible long-term health consequences.

If you determine that you do have food sensitivities, note that adrenal dysfunction can worsen the problem and that food sensitivities can place additional stress on the adrenals, so be sure to consult the section on adrenals in chapter 8. And because food sensitivities can damage the digestive system, also read chapter 5 closely. And as an indication of how intertwined all of these systems are, damage to the digestive system due to food sensitivities can result in nutrient deficiencies, so chapters 7 and 8 may also be relevant for you.

True Food Allergies

Delayed food sensitivities (described next) are more often the cause of mood problems than true food allergies, but since you may be more familiar with true food allergies, or immediate reactions, I'll explain them first. With true food allergies, the food causes the body to make a type of antibody known as IgE (immunoglobulin E). You'll notice an effect within a few minutes of eating the food. For example, if you have a true allergy to shellfish, you could experience throat constriction, watery eyes, itching, and sometimes even asthma or anaphylactic shock, all within a few minutes. True food allergies only affect a small percentage of the population. Foods that commonly cause these severe reactions are wheat, shellfish, eggs, cow's milk, nuts, soy, and white fish (Lipski 2004). If you have IgE allergies to certain foods, you'll need to avoid those foods indefinitely.

Food Sensitivities or Delayed Food Reactions

With delayed food reactions, it may take a few hours to several days before symptoms appear, which can make it difficult to identify the offending food or foods (Lipski 2004). In these reactions, the body responds by creating a type of antibody known as IgG (immunoglobulin G).

In *Digestive Wellness*, clinical nutritionist Elizabeth Lipski (2004) states that 24 percent of American adults claim they have delayed food and environmental reactions. She feels that these sensitivities are often the result of leaky gut syndrome, a condition characterized by damage to the microvilli lining the intestinal walls. This allows undigested food particles to travel across the intestinal wall and into the blood, where the immune system responds to them as foreign, harmful substances and creates antibodies to neutralize them. If you find that you're sensitive to a large number of foods, there's a good chance you have leaky gut syndrome.

Unlike true food allergies, with delayed food reactions almost any food can cause a problem. The foods that most commonly cause reactions are wheat, dairy, eggs, beef, citrus, and pork, which together cause 80 percent of delayed food reactions (Lipski 2004). It doesn't surprise me that beef is a common problem while lamb isn't. Lamb is almost always grass fed, whereas cows are often corn-fed, and I suspect that the corn could be the issue. This is because corn is also a somewhat common problematic food, as are soy, nuts, chocolate, and cane sugar (Pizzorno and Murray 2000). I've also seen problems caused by sensitivities to nightshades (tomatoes, potatoes, eggplant, and peppers), families of foods (such as nuts in general), or foods rich in oxalates (including many leafy greens, nuts, and fruits, as well as wheat, soy, cocoa, black tea, chocolate, and some vegetables).

A delayed food reaction can result in a wide variety of symptoms. In my experience, the top five symptoms are digestive issues, depression and anxiety, low energy, increased cravings, and sleep problems. I've had many clients with a sensitivity to gluten who had wide-ranging symptoms, including mood swings, tension and fear, depression, headaches, nasal congestion, constipation, bloating, indigestion, heartburn, insomnia, skin problems, muscle and joint aches, and fatigue.

Problems with Gluten

Some people are sensitive to a protein called gliadin, which is part of gluten, found in wheat, barley, rye, and various forms of wheat or wheat hybrids, such as spelt, kamut, and triticale. Oats are sometimes excluded from gluten-free diets because of contamination with gluten during processing, but they don't actually contain gluten; instead, they contain avenin, which most people, including many people with celiac disease, can tolerate. But finding certified gluten-free oats is key.

When you hear that someone is having problems with gluten, you may think of digestive problems, such as diarrhea or constipation, abdominal pain, gas, and bloating, and these are indeed common problems caused by gluten. However, gluten can cause much more than just digestive problems.

Gluten, Anxiety, and Other Mood Problems

I've seen so many clients experience dramatic mood improvements when they avoid gluten, so I always recommend that my clients with anxiety and other mood problems go gluten free. Doing so may completely resolve symptoms of anxiety, especially among people who aren't benefiting from antianxiety medications (Potocki and Hozyasz 2002). Clinical experience and specific studies support the connection between gluten and anxiety (Hallert et al. 2009; Pynnönen et al. 2004), social phobia (Addolorato, et al. 2008), depression (Pynnönen et al. 2005), and even schizophrenia (Kalaydjian et al. 2006). Many of the mental health studies have focused on celiac disease, but even if you don't have celiac disease, if you have mood problems or troublesome physical symptoms and avoiding gluten makes a difference, it makes sense to do so.

■ Linda's Story

Linda, a teacher in her late forties, had both mood issues and digestive problems. She found substantial relief from her anxiety by taking GABA, tryptophan, and some basic supplements, like a multivitamin, zinc, and vitamin B_6, but she still had some anxiety and related symptoms. From the start, I recommended that she avoid gluten, but for months she resisted because she loved pizza and was convinced that her made-from-scratch pizza with a whole wheat crust was healthy.

As the months wore on and her symptoms lingered, she finally agreed to try giving up gluten. She was amazed to discover that her anxiety completely dissipated and her lifelong problem with constipation disappeared. If she accidentally ate something with gluten, she knew immediately—she felt nervous and bloated and, eventually, constipated. Because she still loves pizza, she did some research and experimented with making gluten-free crusts. Now she can still enjoy her pizza—and feel great afterward.

Gluten and the Digestive System

Sensitivity to gluten may result in digestive problems like gas, bloating, constipation, or diarrhea. If you have digestive issues in addition to anxiety, it's likely that the microvilli of your intestinal wall are damaged and need time to heal. You may also have nutrient deficiencies as a result of this damage, including low levels of the B vitamins, vitamins A, D, E and K, and iron (which could lead to anemia), as well as tryptophan (Ross 2004). Some of these deficiencies could be contributing to your anxiety symptoms. One study found that supplementing with 800 mcg of folic acid, 500 mcg of vitamin B_{12} (cyanocobalamin), and only 3 mg of vitamin B_6 daily for six months improved the general well-being of people with celiac disease, while also helping with anxiety and depression (Hallert et al. 2009). Bone broths are very healing for the gut, as are glutamine, vitamin C, and aloe vera. For more thorough information on how to support digestive function, consult chapter 5, which addresses this topic in detail.

Testing for Gluten Sensitivities

Specific tests can determine whether gluten is an issue for you, or you can do an elimination-challenge trial, in which you quit eating the potentially problematic food for two weeks to see if symptoms resolve, and then reintroduce it to see if symptoms reappear. Consider doing both. Although seeing test results in print is extremely helpful, testing is not always conclusive and may not indicate you have an issue even if, in fact, you do. Plus, experiencing how much better you feel without problem foods—and how much worse you feel when you reintroduce them—can provide powerful incentive to change your diet.

Two-Week Gluten Elimination-Challenge Trial

You may find the prospect of an elimination-challenge trial daunting. If so, just remind yourself that two weeks is a very short time to give up one specific food, and that the results of this test may help you resolve a variety of mood, digestive, and other health problems.

1. Quit eating all foods that contain gluten for two weeks; this is the elimination phase. As a reminder, foods with gluten include anything containing wheat, rye, barley, spelt, kamut, or triticale. Because oats are frequently contaminated with gluten during processing, eliminate them as well. You can purchase oats labeled gluten free, but I encourage you to avoid even these during the two-week elimination trial. During the elimination period, it's best to eat homemade whole foods, as gluten shows up in many processed foods in the form of ingredients like hydrolyzed protein, textured vegetable protein, and a myriad other derivatives of wheat, rye, and barley, such as barley malt and modified starch. It's in most soy sauces and natural flavorings, and in red wine, beer, and many other fermented beverages. Less obvious sources include the glue on envelopes and fillers in medications and supplements.

2. During the two weeks, observe symptoms related to anxiety, depression, energy, focus, bloating, gas, and constipation, and note any changes. Use the Food, Mood, Energy, Cravings, and Sleep Log (appendix 2) to monitor what you eat and when, how you feel before you eat (tired, hungry, ravenous, needing comfort, and so on), how you feel after you eat (tired, happy, satisfied, comforted, energized, and so on), and bowel movements.

3. On day 15, consume something with gluten at both breakfast and lunch (this is the challenge phase), and then don't eat anything with gluten for three days. I recommend that you choose yeast-free bread for this challenge because yeast may also be a problem, and this

would taint the results of your trial. Try something like yeast-free pancakes or a muffin for breakfast and pasta for lunch.

4. Observe for adverse effects over the course of the next three days, since delayed reactions can take that long to show up. Watch for increased anxiety, moodiness, depression, irritability, fatigue, difficulty focusing, bloating, gas, a change in your bowel movements, or an increase in aches and pains.

If you notice increased symptoms during the challenge phase, you're probably sensitive to gluten. This may be a true allergy, a delayed reaction, or celiac disease. Further testing (described next), can help determine which it is. Or you may not have any increase in symptoms, in which case gluten probably isn't an issue for you. If you aren't certain, you can go off gluten for another two weeks and then challenge again.

As mentioned, a good reason for doing an elimination-challenge trial is that lab tests can be inconclusive or result in false negatives. I once worked with a family, two parents and two children, who all had both anxiety and digestive issues with gluten. Each person tested positive on a different test and negative on others. No matter what your test results, I encourage you to avoid gluten if it affects you adversely.

Lab Tests for Gluten Sensitivity

Lab tests for gluten sensitivity include saliva tests for antigliadin antibodies and blood tests for IgG antibodies and thyroid antibodies. If you have elevated levels of these antibodies, it's cause for concern and indicates that you should avoid gluten and also be tested for celiac disease (Braly and Hoggan 2002). There are other gluten sensitivity markers that aren't currently measured, and they may provide additional useful results in the future.

Salivary Antigliadin Antibodies

Many at-home saliva tests for adrenal function, such as the Adrenal Stress Index (ASI) offered by Diagnos-Techs, include antigliadin antibodies. Many people test positive for antigliadin antibodies. The ASI also includes secretory immunoglobulin (SIgA), an antibody that plays a critical role in immunity in the gastrointestinal tract. When testing antigliadin antibodies, it's important to also measure levels of SIgA; if levels of SIgA are low, it may cause a false negative result for antigliadin antibodies. SIgA is often low as a result of stress and adrenal fatigue. Many other labs, including Metametrix, also measure both antigliadin antibodies and SIgA in various saliva and stool tests.

IgG Antibodies for Gluten-Containing Grains

Delayed reactions to foods (IgG food sensitivities) can be identified by blood tests that require either a blood (serum) draw or a finger prick. Known as an enzyme-linked immunosorbent assay (ELISA), this type of testing can be very effective (Atkinson et al. 2004; Shakib et al. 2006), especially when considered in conjunction with your symptoms and health history and a food log (Pizzorno and Murray 2000). ELISA testing will indicate if your body is having an immune reaction to various foods, including wheat, rye, barley, and oats, and whether specific foods are causing a mild, medium, or strong reaction.

If testing indicates that you're experiencing delayed food reactions, I recommend that you remove any problem foods for at least three months, and then reintroduce them one by one, waiting at least three days after adding each one before adding the next. If you experience any symptoms during those three days, you may need to avoid that food indefinitely. If you don't experience renewed symptoms, it's probably fine to eat that food on a rotational basis (every third day or so).

Metametrix Labs offers two tests that check for delayed reactions to grains with gluten, as well as other foods: Allergix IgG4 Food Antibodies 90–Serum, which assesses reactions to ninety foods people are often sensitive to, and Allergix IgG4 Food Antibodies–Bloodspot 30, which assesses reactions to thirty foods.

Elevated Thyroid Antibodies

Elevated levels of two thyroid antibodies—antithyroglobulin and antithyroperoxidase—may indicate that you have Hashimoto's thyroiditis, in which the body is creating antibodies to its own thyroid gland. This autoimmune condition is common among people with celiac disease (Naiyer et al. 2008; Barker and Liu 2008) or gluten sensitivity. Levels of both antibodies can be assessed with blood tests that your doctor can order. If your levels are elevated, avoiding gluten completely and taking 200 mcg of selenium daily may help normalize your thyroid function and lower levels of thyroid antibodies.

Testing for Celiac Disease

Two tests can help you determine whether you have celiac disease. One is a simple blood test; the other is a biopsy. IgE and gene testing are other options, as is testing for elevated thyroid antibodies (mentioned previously), which is common in celiac disease.

The Celiac Profile, a blood test from Metametrix, measures the following three markers of celiac disease, however negative results don't completely rule out gluten sensitivity or celiac disease:

- IgA tissue transglutaminase (IgA-tTG): Elevated levels identify about 98 percent of those with celiac disease (Braly and Hoggan 2002).

- IgA antigliadin antibodies (IgA-AGA): Elevated levels indicate a reaction against gliadin, which also indicates the diet isn't gluten free.

- Serum IgA: Low levels indicate a ten to fifteen times greater risk for developing celiac disease and can also result in a false negative result for IgA-tTG.

The medical community generally considers biopsy of the small intestine to be the gold standard for diagnosing celiac disease. If the biopsy shows flattened microvilli, the patient is encouraged to adopt a gluten-free diet. If a second biopsy, done after the person follows a gluten-free diet for some time, shows improvement, celiac disease is diagnosed. However, there are limitations to this method (Braly and Hoggan 2002). Biopsies can miss damage because it can vary from one area to another or vary over time. And if a person with celiac disease has avoided gluten for more than a few weeks, the gut may have healed, so there will be no damage.

If neither of these tests indicates celiac disease but you think you may be sensitive to gluten, there are a couple of other tests you may want to consider. Test for the genes HLA-DQ2 and HLA-DQ8, as both are associated with a greater risk of having celiac disease, as well as other autoimmune diseases, including type 1 diabetes and autoimmune thyroid disease (Barker and Liu 2008). However, people without celiac disease may also carry these genes (Braly and Hoggan 2002), so results aren't definitive. Your doctor can order these tests, or EnteroLab offers this genetic testing via an at-home kit. The benefit of genetic testing is that it can provide an early indication that you may have problems with gluten, before positive results are seen on some of the other tests.

Alternatives to Grains That Contain Gluten

If gluten is a problem for you, you can still eat rice, corn, buckwheat, quinoa, amaranth, and probably oats (if they're certified gluten free). Although millet doesn't contain gluten, some people have problems with it. You'll have to experiment and see for yourself. Thankfully, there's growing awareness of the potential problems with gluten, and these days you can find gluten-free versions of a wide variety of grain-based foods—bread, pasta, crackers, waffles, and more. These foods are made with a wide variety of alternative flours, made from rice, corn, potatoes, various beans, and even coconut. There are also many wonderful gluten-free cookbooks, but some call for excessive sugar or other less-than-healthful ingredients. Before purchasing a gluten-free cookbook, review it closely, keeping your dietary needs and the recommendations in chapters 1 and 2 in mind. You'll also find many great online resources for information and gluten-free products.

However, rather than simply replacing the problem grains with another grain (for example, replacing wheat pasta with rice pasta), consider incorporating more vegetables into your diet. Starchy vegetables like sweet potato, squash, and carrots are a wonderfully nutritious source of carbohydrates, vitamins, and minerals.

If you have trouble with gluten but don't have celiac disease, certain preparation methods may help your body handle gluten better. Many traditional diets include soaked or fermented grains, as in sourdough bread. These methods help make grains more digestible and possibly less of an issue for mood problems, digestive issues, or both. There is some evidence that sourdough bread can be tolerated by those with gluten sensitivity, including people with celiac disease (Di Cagno et al. 2004). However, it's best to err on the side of caution. If you experiment with these foods, see how you feel, then base your decision on your experience. It can be helpful to take an enzyme supplement that will help you digest the proteins in gluten (as well as casein). That way, if you do consume something with gluten by mistake, the ill effects will be lessened. Look for a supplement containing the enzyme dipeptidyl peptidase IV (DPP IV).

If Gluten Isn't a Problem

Even if you can tolerate gluten, it's still important to avoid processed grains such as white flour and foods made from it, including cookies, cake, white pasta, and so on. Whole grain products are always a better choice. Sprouted whole grain bread is another good option. I still recommend not making them a staple of your diet, and definitely don't eat gluten-containing grains at every meal.

Problems with Dairy Consumption

The gluten problems that are so common with anxiety and mood issues can damage the gut lining and result in problems with dairy consumption. It's important to address this to prevent further damage to the digestive system and potential nutrient deficiencies. This kind of problem with dairy may disappear after the gut heals.

Dairy doesn't cause anxiety per se, but the increased mucus production, damage to the digestive system, and immune response can have indirect impacts on mood.

Some people lack the enzyme lactase, which digests lactose, the sugar in dairy products (Bolin 2009). This affects about 75 percent of people worldwide (Lipski 2004). Dairy can have a similar opiate-like effect as gluten, giving you a psychological high followed by a letdown. Think about how you feel before and after eating a big bowl of ice cream. Is it a comfort food? If eating it feels like a big reward, and then later you feel ill, tired, and congested, you may be addicted to it.

Because issues with dairy are so common, I encourage you to do a two-week dairy elimination-challenge trial, even if you doubt it will make a difference. You can also use IgG testing to identify delayed reactions to dairy (Shakib et al. 2006). If you find you can tolerate dairy, follow the guidelines in chapter 1.

Problems with Other Foods

Potentially, any food can result in a delayed food reaction, and as mentioned, for some people this can be a factor in anxiety due to gut damage and nutrient deficiencies, as well as stressing the adrenals. A study of people with irritable bowel syndrome used IgG antibody testing to identify problem foods. Removing those foods led to significant improvements in symptoms, as well as improved quality of life and reduced anxiety and depression (Atkinson et al. 2004). The patients who best complied with their dietary restrictions experienced the greatest improvements. When the restrictions were relaxed, many symptoms returned.

If you still suspect food is an issue but don't have a problem with gluten or dairy (or if you do but removing them doesn't completely resolve your symptoms), you can identify other food sensitivities with IgG testing. The IgG tests available from Metametrix Labs (described previously for gluten) also check for reactions to many other common foods. If IgG testing indicates that many different foods are causing a reaction, leaky gut syndrome may be the issue. You need to avoid all of the problematic foods and let the gut heal.

You can also do the elimination-challenge trial (as described previously) with any foods that you suspect may be causing problems, or with the remaining foods that most commonly cause problems: beef, citrus, eggs, pork, corn, soy, nuts, chocolate, and cane sugar. If you have favorite foods that you eat all the time, these would be worth investigating too. I had one client who ate strawberries and almonds every single day, and both proved to be a problem for her.

Finally, if your results are unclear and you have a strong suspicion that some food is causing problems for you, you could follow the hypoallergenic or oligoantigenic diet. With this approach, you eat only those foods that are least likely to cause problems, typically brown rice, lamb, all fruit except citrus, and all vegetables except tomatoes, eggplant, peppers, and potatoes. After eating only these foods for two weeks, you can add a new food back into your diet every three days and watch for reactions (Pizzorno and Murray 2000). A German study of children with hyperactivity and disruptive behavior disorder found that this approach improved the behavior of about 25 percent of the children (Schmidt et al. 1997).

Problems with All Grains, Starchy Vegetables, and Legumes

If you feel moody, anxious, tired, or restless after eating any grains (rice, corn, and so on), starchy vegetables (potatoes, sweet potatoes, and so on), or legumes, then it's possible that these carbohydrates are not being digested and instead are fermenting and feeding harmful bacteria in your digestive system. If this is the case, it's worth doing an elimination-challenge trial and following the Specific Carbohydrate Diet (SCD) guidelines. The SCD, which became well-known with the publication of *Breaking the Vicious Cycle* (2002), by Elaine Gottschall, helps with digestive problems like Crohn's disease, colitis, and chronic diarrhea, as well as mood problems, including anxiety and depression.

With the SCD, specific carbohydrates are allowed. Fruits can be eaten, but not starchy vegetables (potatoes, sweet potatoes), grains (all gluten-containing grains, as well as rice, corn, millet, and other gluten-free grains), or legumes. Other than fruit, the following are allowed: meat, fish, chicken, eggs, nuts, and nonstarchy vegetables such as green beans, asparagus, cauliflower, broccoli, and so on. Fats and oils such as butter, olive oil, and coconut oil are permitted.

Natasha Campbell-McBride, author of *Gut and Psychology Syndrome* (GAPS; 2008), has taken this diet one step further and added healing bone broths and fermented foods, based on the traditional food concepts of the Weston A. Price Foundation. Freshly squeezed vegetable juices for detoxification and probiotic supplements are also allowed. Campbell-McBride reports huge successes with anxiety, depression, bipolar disorder, autism, arthritis, and many learning disorders, as well as digestive complaints. She has her patients eat this way for a year or longer.

Although not specifically referring to the SCD/GAPS diet, in one study (Austin et al. 2009) a very low carbohydrate diet (20 grams per day, or only 4 percent carbohydrate) was shown to be beneficial for irritable bowel syndrome, and as you'll read in chapter 5, anxiety is common with irritable bowel syndrome. Another study (King, Elia, and Hunter 1998) also found that people with irritable bowel syndrome have abnormal colonic fermentation of carbohydrates.

If you decide to follow the SCD or GAPS diet, I suggest not relying quite so heavily on nuts and nut flours for baking. First, nuts can be a problem if you have a nut allergy or sensitivity. Additionally, nuts have a higher copper to zinc ratio, and too many can potentially result in elevated copper levels, which is not good for anxiety (refer to chapter 7, on zinc and vitamin B_6).

I have only had a small number of clients who needed to eat the SCD/GAPS way, but for those who have problems with all grains and starchy vegetables, the improvements are profound. This diet is also very beneficial if you have candida overgrowth, a bacterial imbalance, or parasites (see chapter 5).

Overview of Various Types of Food Sensitivity That May Affect Anxiety or Mood					
	True food allergy	Food sensitivity	Gluten sensitivity	Celiac disease	SCD/GAPS
Anxiety and depression	Not common	Sometimes	Common	Common	Common
Ages	Mostly children	All ages	All ages	All ages	All ages
Testing	IgE mediated	Nonimmunological or IgG, elimination trial	Thyroid antibodies, IgG, SIgA, antigliadin antibodies, HLA–DQ genes, elimination trial	Thyroid antibodies, IgA-tTG, SIgA, IgA-AGA, antigliadin antibodies, biopsy, HLA-DQ genes, elimination trial	Elimination trial, stool tests
Foods	Few	Many	Gluten-containing grains	Gluten-containing grains	All grains and starchy vegetables
Reaction timing	Immediate	Delayed	Delayed	Delayed	Delayed
Types of reaction	Usually the same, often physical	Variable, both physical and mental	Variable, both physical and mental	Variable, both physical and mental	Variable, both physical and mental
Diagnosis	Straightforward	Often obscure	Difficult	Difficult	Difficult

Using Amino Acids to Reduce Cravings

In *The Diet Cure* (2011), Julia Ross suggests using targeted amino acids to help reduce cravings and make it easier to avoid problem foods, especially carbohydrates, such as baked goods, breads, and other grains, as well as dairy and sweets. This approach has been extremely helpful for the majority of my clients, often within minutes of taking the amino acid. Here are some examples:

- If you have afternoon or evening cravings for carbohydrates and gluten-containing grains, you may have low serotonin. Tryptophan or 5-hydroxytryptophan may help.

- If you crave comfort foods, like bread, cookies, or ice cream, they may be providing an endorphin rush. Taking D-phenylalanine (DPA) may help.

- If you overeat bread, cereal, pasta, or dairy to calm down, you may have low levels of GABA. Taking supplemental GABA may help you relax and experience fewer anxiety-related cravings.

- If you're prone to low blood sugar and have intense cravings for something sweet or starchy, glutamine really helps, as it plays a role in moderating blood sugar levels.

- If you crave something sweet for a quick energy fix, you may have low levels of catecholamines. Taking supplemental tyrosine may help.

Glutamine is covered in chapter 2, and the other amino acids are discussed in chapter 6. Before supplementing with amino acids, be sure to read chapter 6 closely, especially the section "Amino Acid Precautions."

■ Susan's Story

Susan, a thirty-one-year-old stay-at-home mother of three, had been suffering from worsening eczema for ten years.

Her flare-ups had become increasingly unpleasant and were starting to affect her mood, her sleep, and, as she reported, her sanity. She was on medication for depression and had a problem with anxiety and terrible sugar cravings. Her diet was full of cookies, cakes, candies, and sugar in a variety of other forms. In an attempt to control her eczema, she'd been using Benadryl daily for over ten years and had also tried cortisone creams and a wide range of other common treatments, but nothing helped. Her eczema had gotten so painful that she wasn't able to shower. And although Susan had been a competitive gymnast in her twenties and loved to exercise, she hadn't been able to because even the sweat on her skin was too painful.

All of her symptoms were driving her crazy, but it was the ugly and uncomfortable rashes around her eyes and on her chin, neck, and arms that finally motivated her to work with a nutritionist and try something new. At my recommendation, she agreed to stop eating gluten for a two-week trial. She also supplemented with specific amino acids: D-phenylalanine (DPA) to help with her comfort-related food cravings, glutamine to help with blood sugar control, and GABA to help with her anxiety. There was no change in her skin during the first week, but because of the amino acids her cravings for sugary foods diminished substantially, which helped her improve her diet a lot during that first week. She started eating plenty of vegetables and high-quality protein and had a breakfast smoothie every day and olive oil on her salads.

During our second appointment, we figured out that there was wheat in the whey protein powder she was using in her breakfast smoothie. She replaced it with whey that was gluten free, so during week two, her diet was truly gluten free. The results were nothing short of dramatic. Her eczema virtually disappeared, and for the first time in ages, she was sleeping through the night. During that second week, she took Benadryl only once and was able to shower each day. She didn't really even need amino acids long term. She started taking less GABA and was eager to talk to her doctor about stopping her antidepressant medications—because she no longer felt depressed!

We also tested her reactions to gluten. Despite her many symptoms, all of the gluten-related tests came back negative, but she was feeling so much better that she decided to continue avoiding gluten anyway.

By the third week, she was starting to plan an exercise program and was thrilled about that. What a change in just a few short weeks. Susan said, "I feel better than I have in ten years. I feel I can do anything again. This is me! I am so, so happy!" I checked in with her a few months later, and although her eczema still wasn't completely healed, it was under control. In addition, she had been able to quit taking antidepressants, had lost over ten pounds, was working again, and was free from both anxiety and depression.

Allergies and Anxiety Due to Low Blood Histamine

As mentioned, histamine also functions as a neurotransmitter and can therefore also have an impact on mood, resulting in paranoia, phobias, OCD, and depression, in addition to physical symptoms, including food and environmental allergies. Although histamine imbalances have been researched (Braverman and Weissberg 1987; Jackson et al. 1998) and successfully treated in clinical settings (Pfeiffer 1987; Mathews-Larson 2001), it still isn't common practice to assess for histamine imbalances in relation to mood disorders. Whole blood histamine testing is offered by Health Diagnostics and Research Institute. In *Depression-Free, Naturally* (2001), nutritionist Joan Mathews-Larson covers the symptoms of low and high histamine, and how to resolve either imbalance. Please consult her excellent book for more details.

How Quickly You Can Expect Improvements

If you have delayed reactions (IgG) to any foods, you can probably expect to see improvements in mood or digestive symptoms within three days of removing them from your diet. (After three months you can consider trying to reintroduce excluded foods.)

If you have immediate reactions (IgE) or have tested positive for celiac disease, you can expect improvements as soon as you remove problematic foods from your diet. You'll have to avoid these foods indefinitely.

If you have problems with grains and starchy vegetables, you can expect some improvements within a few weeks of removing these foods from your diet, but it can take twelve months or longer for symptoms to completely resolve.

It typically takes three months to correct histamine imbalances.

In all cases, the time frame may differ from person to person, and it will also vary depending on how strict you are about avoiding problem foods. So it really depends on you and your unique biochemistry, as well as the time it takes for your gut to heal.

CHAPTER 5

Improve Your Digestion

Digestive disorders are very common in the United States. Over a third of all adults are affected, and each year forty-five million people visit the doctor for reflux, constipation, irritable bowel syndrome (IBS), liver disease, and other digestive complaints (Burt and Schappert 2004; Adams, Hendershot, and Marano 1999). Studies have found that people with digestive complaints such as IBS, food allergies and sensitivities, small intestinal bacterial overgrowth, and ulcerative colitis frequently suffer from anxiety and, to a lesser extent, depression (Addolorato, et al. 2008). One study (Lydiard 2001) found that 50 to 90 percent of people with IBS who visited a doctor for treatment also suffered from various anxiety disorders (panic disorder, generalized anxiety disorder, social phobia, and post-traumatic stress disorder) and major depression.

It can be difficult to assess which came first. Is the anxiety affecting your digestion, or did poor digestion lead to anxiety or make anxiety worse? Sometimes it's a mixture of both, and both need to be addressed. Can you relate to the following phrases? "I have butterflies in my stomach," "I can feel it in my gut," or "I just have this awful feeling in the pit of my stomach." These aren't just figures of speech. According to Dr. Michael Gershon in his groundbreaking book *The Second Brain* (1998), all of the neurotransmitters that are found in the brain are also found in the digestive system—hence the term "second brain." The digestive system actually has its own nervous system and over 95 percent of serotonin is made in the gut (Gershon 1998). A study looking at people with chronic fatigue syndrome and an imbalance in intestinal bacteria supports this gut-brain-mood connection, finding that those treated with probiotics not only had greater numbers of beneficial bacteria, but also had a significant decrease in anxiety and depression (Rao et al. 2009).

There is much to be said for the concept that all disease begins in the gut. I'm sure you've heard the expression, "You are what you eat." If you eat healthful food, you will be healthy—or much more likely to be healthy (and if you eat unhealthful food, you're much more likely to be unhealthy)—at least up to a point. If you eat wholesome, nutrient-dense food but can't effectively digest and absorb what you eat, you won't be healthy. For optimal health, including mental stability and good immunity, you need to have a healthy digestive system.

In this chapter, I'll provide a brief description of the digestive process, outline a few of the many causes of poor digestion, and help you explore how you can improve your digestion. Because there are so many topics to be covered in this book as a whole, I can only provide an overview of issues with digestion—just enough to give you an awareness of what to consider. For more detailed information, I recommend Elizabeth Lipski's wonderful book *Digestive Wellness* (2004).

And in addition to the issues covered in this chapter, be sure to consider other factors that may affect your digestion. For example, a sluggish thyroid can contribute to constipation (see chapter 8); food sensitivities can cause digestive distress and damage (see chapter 4); and low serotonin can affect your digestion (see chapter 6), as can low zinc (see chapter 7), low magnesium (see chapter 8), and adrenal fatigue (see chapter 8). As always, a wholesome diet (covered in chapter 1) is vital. And if you eat large amounts of sugar, it can feed candida and make digestive issues worse (see chapter 2 for more on sugar). Stress also plays an important role; if this is an issue for you, consider some of the lifestyle changes outlined in chapter 8.

Poor Digestion Questionnaire

This questionnaire will help you identify if you have digestive problems and what might be causing them. It's divided into clusters of symptoms related to different potential causes. With any of these causes, anxiety, depression, or mood swings could occur as a result. Check off any of the following symptoms or signs that apply to you on a regular basis:

Low Levels of Stomach Acid

☐ Excessive burping, bloating, or gas immediately after meals

☐ Feeling overly full during and immediately after meals

☐ Having intestinal parasites, candida overgrowth, or dysbiosis

☐ Indigestion, constipation, diarrhea, or difficult bowel movements

☐ Getting an upset stomach or nausea easily after taking supplements

☐ Having undigested foods in your stool

☐ Having multiple food sensitivities, food allergies, or celiac disease

☐ Having iron deficiency or low levels of zinc

Low Levels of Pancreatic Enzymes

☐ Fatigue, indigestion, or excessive fullness for one to three hours after eating

☐ Stomachaches or pain, tenderness, and soreness on your left side under your rib cage

☐ Gas or bloating

☐ Constipation or diarrhea, with fiber causing constipation

☐ Nausea or vomiting

☐ Stool containing undigested food or being foul smelling, mucuslike, greasy, shiny, or poorly formed

Large Intestine Issues

☐ Feeling that your bowel does not empty completely

☐ Pain in the lower abdomen that's relieved by passing stool or gas, or having large amounts of foul-smelling gas

☐ Constipation, diarrhea, or alternating constipation and diarrhea

☐ Hard, dry, or small stool

☐ Coated tongue

☐ Having more than three bowel movements daily

☐ Using laxatives frequently

Bacterial Imbalance or Parasites

☐ Chronic constipation or diarrhea

☐ Itchy ears, nose, or anus

☐ Restlessness or grinding your teeth at night, waking often, or night sweats

☐ Food sensitivities or allergies

☐ Low energy, fatigue, or joint or muscle aches and pains

☐ Hives, rashes, eczema, skin ulcers, or sores

☐ Dark circles under your eyes or wrinkles around your mouth

Candida Overgrowth

☐ Nail or skin fungus, athlete's foot, or vaginal yeast infection

☐ Chronic sinus or ear infections

☐ Food sensitivities

☐ Feeling chronically fatigued

☐ Poor memory and focus

☐ Constipation or diarrhea

☐ Frequent bloating and gas

☐ Cravings for bread, cookies, sugar, other carbohydrates, or alcohol

Liver or Gallbladder Problems

☐ Sensitivity to greasy or high-fat foods

☐ Lower bowel gas or bloating several hours after eating

☐ Sour or metallic taste in the mouth

☐ Itchy skin or yellowish whites of the eyes

☐ Stool color alternates from clay colored to normal brown

☐ Bad breath or bad body odor

☐ History of gallbladder attacks or stones or gallbladder removal

If you checked off more than three items in any area, the next sections will help you improve your digestion. This questionnaire is based on my experience working with many clients, along with information from *Digestive Wellness* (2004), by Elizabeth Lipski, and *Textbook of Natural Medicine* (2000), by Joseph Pizzorno and Michael Murray.

The Digestive Process

Assimilating nutrients from the food you eat is a two-part process consisting of digestion and absorption. Strictly speaking, digestion refers to breaking down food into smaller units that can be absorbed by the body. The process of digestion is both mechanical and chemical. The mechanical aspects include chewing, churning of food in the stomach, and mixing it with enzymes and digestive juices, which accomplish the chemical process, breaking down large food molecules into smaller particles.

Carbohydrate digestion starts in the mouth, with saliva, but most of it is accomplished in the small intestine by pancreatic and other enzymes. Carbohydrates are broken down into glucose. Protein digestion starts in the stomach with gastric acid (primarily hydrochloric acid) and the enzyme pepsin. Protein digestion is also completed in the small intestine by pancreatic and other enzymes. Proteins are broken down into amino acids. Fat digestion is accomplished mostly in the small intestine by pancreatic enzymes and by bile, which is produced by the liver and stored in the gallbladder. Fats are broken down into fatty acids and glycerol.

Once the food you eat has been broken down, its nutrients are absorbed through the intestinal wall and transferred into the blood and lymph, which circulate them to your cells for energy and healing. Nutrients and water are absorbed from the small intestine, and some water is also absorbed from the large intestine.

Why Good Digestion and Absorption Are Important

Good digestion and absorption are important for a number of reasons. Here are a few of them:

- They allow your cells to use the glucose, amino acids, and fatty acids—the building blocks of carbohydrates, proteins, and fats.

- These processes also make available all of the vitamins, minerals, antioxidants, and other nutrients that nature has so beautifully packaged into healthful whole foods. Your long-term mental and physical health is dependent on a continual supply of these nutrients, which are used to make enzymes, hormones, and neurotransmitters, and to aid in all of the body's physiological processes.

- They will protect you from parasites, imbalanced intestinal bacteria, and candida overgrowth, all of which can further compromise your digestion and often disrupt mood and sleep and intensify cravings.

- The body makes much of its serotonin in the gut, as well as some of its B vitamins, so having a healthy digestive system is important for adequate levels of these mood-boosting compounds.

Using Your Stool as a Clue to Your Digestive Function

Your stool can give you a big clue about your digestion. It should be well formed, shaped like a banana, soft like a ripe banana, and well-hydrated and slippery (Lewis and Heaton 1997). It shouldn't be light colored, but rather a chocolate-brown color. You shouldn't need a laxative, you should be able to eliminate easily without straining, and you should have a bowel movement at least once a day. Having two or three well-formed bowel movements is fine too.

Eating Guidelines for Good Digestion

We live in a fast-paced world, we often eat on the run, and many of us rely on processed foods. Take a few minutes to consider these questions:

- Do you eat on the run, eat in front of the TV, or not sit down to eat?

- Do you eat when you're under high stress?

- Do you tend to eat fast foods or processed foods?

- Do you eat few or no fresh vegetables or fruit, or eat a diet low in fiber?

- Do you drink less than 2 quarts (64 fluid ounces) of water a day?

If this sounds like you, just improving your eating habits can make a huge difference, preventing or helping resolve digestive problems, and also enhancing mood and overall health. If the following suggestions don't help your digestion, you'll need to investigate other potential problems, such as low levels of stomach acid, large-intestine issues, bacterial imbalances, and candida overgrowth.

Eat Foods That Promote Good Digestion and Skip Poor-Quality Food

Western cultures tend to eat fewer of the foods that promote good digestion. If you eat poor-quality, refined, processed foods, this will affect your digestion. It's important to follow the eating guidelines in chapter 1, with a focus on specific foods when your digestion tends to be sluggish. Here are some tips on foods that can be helpful:

- Raw foods are full of enzymes, which can aid digestion. Eat plenty of leafy greens, snack on raw vegetables, and add raw vegetables, such as carrots, zucchini, and celery, to salads.

- Fermented or cultured foods and beverages contain probiotics, or beneficial bacteria, which make these foods more digestible and enhance digestion. Some examples are yogurt, kefir, sauerkraut, kimchi, and kombucha.

- Bitter foods such as arugula and dandelion greens stimulate the production of the body's own digestive enzymes.

- Soaked grains and nuts and sprouted beans and seeds are more digestible and more nutrient dense.

Change Your Eating Habits

While choosing the right foods can lead to big improvements in digestion, it's also important to consider your eating habits. Here are some tips in this regard:

Prepare and eat your meals at home. Food preparation should be fun and enjoyable, not a chore. Get the whole family involved and try new recipes. Thinking about the meal, seeing the food, and smelling the aromas during preparation all prepare your body for digestion, getting your digestive juices and enzymes flowing in advance of eating (Feldman and Richardson 1986). Just think about how your saliva starts to flow when you smell a pot of stew cooking.

Chew your food well. The digestive process starts in the mouth, so chewing your food well is important. It breaks foods into smaller pieces and mixes them with salivary enzymes.

Eat smaller meals. Don't overeat. Eating smaller meals, perhaps more frequently, will help you avoid overburdening your digestive system. Don't eat a very large meal late at night, so you can properly digest your food before you go to bed.

Give thanks for your food, savor the meal, and be mindful. Give thanks, say a prayer, or do a blessing. Slow down and savor the flavors, the textures, the aromas, and the experience of eating. Be mindful and think about the food you're eating. I once did a mindfulness exercise where we were guided through the experience of eating a single raisin over the course of five minutes. It is something that will stay with me always. First we looked at the raisin, then we touched it and smelled it. Then we put it in our mouths and very, very slowly chewed it, attending to its texture, juices, and sweetness. This is such a contrast to the way we usually gulp our food down.

Sit down to eat, and make it a family gathering. Definitely sit down to eat, and eat at the table with family and friends, not in front of the TV. Keep the conversation positive and light. I love this idea offered by fellow nutritionist and good friend Robin Nielsen: she suggests that just lighting a candle can be calming and put you in a digestive mode. In *The New Whole Foods Encyclopedia* (1999), Rebecca Wood offers this suggestion for feeling less alone when you eat by yourself: remove extra chairs from the table and put photos of loved ones nearby where you can see them.

Don't eat when you're highly stressed or anxious. Chronic stress, anxiety, and depression reduce your production of hydrochloric acid and lower levels of secretory immunoglobulin A (SIgA), an antibody that plays a critical role in immunity in the gastrointestinal tract. This will impair your digestion. And because poor digestion leads to nutrient depletions that make it more difficult to handle stress, it creates a vicious cycle. If you need to eat and do feel stressed or anxious, take a few minutes to breathe deeply or practice other relaxation techniques before your meal. Also consider listening to relaxing music while you eat. If you find that you're eating to calm down, and especially if you're eating sugary foods, chapter 2, on sugar, and chapter 6, on brain chemistry, will be very helpful.

Causes of Poor Digestion and How to Improve Your Digestion

In addition to eating poor-quality food and eating on the run, there are a number of physiological reasons why your digestion may be less than ideal. Most of them boil down to a few root causes: low levels of stomach acid or pancreatic enzymes, problems with the large intestine, bacterial imbalance, and candida overgrowth. All are discussed next. In addition, many medications have gastrointestinal side effects. For example, antacids and proton pump inhibitors (like Prilosec) affect protein digestion (Lipski 2004), antibiotics can disrupt your bacterial balance, and pain medications can damage the lining of the digestive system.

Low Levels of Stomach Acid or Pancreatic Enzymes

Low levels of hydrochloric acid (HCl), a condition known as hypochlorhydria, impairs the body's ability break down proteins and therefore limits the availability of tryptophan and other amino acids. This can contribute to depression (Cater 1992), anxiety, sleep problems, and sugar cravings. HCl is also necessary for absorption of vitamin C, the B vitamins (especially vitamin B_{12}), iron, calcium, manganese, and zinc. Sufficient stomach acid also provides your first defense against food poisoning, parasites, bacterial overgrowth, and infections.

Low levels of pancreatic enzymes can impair digestion of protein, fats, and carbohydrates. Both low HCl and low pancreatic enzymes can also contribute to food allergies (Pizzorno and Murray 2000). This is discussed in detail in chapter 4.

Testing for Low Stomach Acid and Pancreatic Enzymes

Certain blood tests may indicate the possibility of low HCl: high or low levels of total serum protein, globulin, and blood urea nitrogen (BUN). All are included in a standard comprehensive metabolic panel.

Stool testing can be helpful in detecting low levels of pancreatic enzymes, indicating whether you have undigested fats and carbohydrates and measuring levels of elastase, an indictor of pancreatic function. Metametrix offers a stool test called the GI Effects Complete Profile, which measures these and also assesses for bacterial imbalances, parasites, and candida overgrowth.

How to Correct Low Stomach Acid or Low Pancreatic Enzymes

If you have low stomach acid or suspect that you do, you can take supplemental betaine HCl. Start with one capsule (typically about 650 mg, which is equivalent to about 10 grains) with each meal, and slowly increase to a maximum of five per meal. If you experience a warmth in your stomach at any one meal, cut back by one capsule and stay with this dose. You may find you need to continue to supplement with HCl, especially as you get older. But you may also find that you need less as your body starts to make its own HCl, so continue to cut back by one capsule anytime you feel a burning sensation (Lipski 2004; Pizzorno and Murray 2000).

Apple cider vinegar may help increase your own HCl production. Try mixing 1 tablespoon in 8 ounces (1 cup) of water and drinking this before each meal. Another way to increase your body's production of HCl is to eat bitter greens, such as arugula and dandelion, before a meal. In Europe, Swedish bitters are a common remedy for low HCl (Lipski 2004). One possible reason for low HCl is a low-salt diet. The chloride in the salt (or sodium chloride) is used to make HCl. Use unrefined salt (see chapter 1).

To compensate for low pancreatic enzymes, you can try taking an enzyme supplement (with or without HCl) containing pancreatic enzymes such as protease, which digests protein; lipase, which digests fats; and amylase, which digests carbohydrates (Lipski 2004). Enzyme products often also contain bromelain (a protease derived from pineapple) and papain (a protease derived from papaya). The dosage is typically 350 to 1,000 mg at each meal (Pizzorno and Murray 2000). If you have problems with wheat or dairy, look for an enzyme supplement containing dipeptidyl peptidase IV (DPP IV), which helps digest the proteins in gluten and casein (Hausch et al. 2002).

Large Intestine Issues

Problems with the large intestine often result in constipation (and sometimes diarrhea). Because the large intestine must store waste until it's excreted, it's important to have regular bowel movements. Eating enough fiber, drinking enough water, having good bowel habits, and various other approaches can all help keep your large intestine functioning well.

Eat enough fiber. Make sure you eat plenty of vegetables and whole grains, such as brown rice, so you get enough fiber. You may also need supplemental fiber. Try mixing 1 tablespoon of psyllium seeds or freshly ground flaxseeds into a smoothie or water once or twice a day.

Drink enough water, but not during meals. Drink enough water (at least 2 quarts, or 64 fluid ounces daily) but don't drink water or other beverages during meals, as this can dilute your digestive enzymes. Your body absorbs water from the large intestine, so if you don't drink enough, your stool will become dry and hard, leading to constipation.

Improve poor bowel habits. It's important that you don't delay going to the bathroom. When you do, water continues to be absorbed from your stool, so it gets hard and dry (Lipski 2004). Also allow time for a satisfactory and complete bowel movement.

Additional solutions for constipation. If you've tried all of the previous recommendations and still have constipation, try eating prunes or drinking prune juice, taking magnesium oxide supplements, or drinking aloe vera juice. Also, have your thyroid assessed, as constipation is common with an underactive thyroid. Massage and exercise can also be helpful.

Bacterial Imbalance or Parasites

Dysbiosis is any imbalance of intestinal bacteria, parasites or, candida. The digestive system hosts both beneficial and harmful, opportunistic bacteria. Sufficient levels of beneficial bacteria prevent overgrowth of harmful bacteria and candida and prevent parasites from taking up residence. Dysbiosis can be caused by low stomach acid (Cater 1992), stress, medications such as antibiotics, poor immunity going into surgery, poor nutrition, or eating a lot of sugar or processed foods (Lipski 2004; Hawrelak and Myers 2004). It can also be caused by poor function of the ileocecal valve, which lies between the small and large intestines. The pressure of strained bowel movements due to constipation can allow the ileocecal valve to remain open, permitting contents of the colon to move back up into the small intestine, disrupting its balance of flora. This ileocecal valve dysfunction is often described as a fluttering feeling in the lower abdomen area. An adjustment in this area by a chiropractor or osteopath can often correct the problem (Lipski 2004).

With dysbiosis, foods may be poorly digested. Undigested food feeds the bad bacteria, perpetuating the imbalance and, ultimately, damaging the digestive lining and leading to leaky gut syndrome (also known as intestinal permeability), a condition in which undigested foods pass through the intestinal wall. This results in food sensitivities because the body sees these particles, particularly proteins, as foreign. The resulting immune response causes inflammation and further damage and malabsorption, creating a vicious cycle of ongoing digestive problems. Dysbiosis can cause mood problems (Crook 1997), including anxiety (Uspenskii and Balukova 2009), as well as arthritis, chronic fatigue, and irritable bowel syndrome (Lipski 2004).

I'll discuss candida at length next, but first I'll briefly address parasites, which are more common than you may think. Certain factors can increase the odds of having them: third-world travel, going barefoot outside, eating sushi or raw meat, having pets, allowing pets to eat from your plate, cleaning up cat litter, drinking untreated water from lakes and streams, and swimming in lakes and rivers. Certain herbs can be used to treat parasites, such as wormwood and black walnut hull, or it may be more effective to work with your doctor and take medications.

Candida Overgrowth

The most prevalent form of dybiosis is intestinal candida overgrowth (also known as yeast or fungal infections). Candida is commonly present in the gastrointestinal tract with no ill effects, but when it becomes invasive, it can cause a host of issues. And, of course, yeast infections can occur in various parts of the body.

Candida overgrowth is usually triggered by antibiotic use, birth control pills, steroid medications, and sugar consumption (Lipski 2004; Crook 1997). Many in the conventional medical community don't see it as a problem that requires treatment, and even fewer see it as contributing to mood issues, but as part of a holistic plan to alleviate anxiety, it must be addressed. I've seen many clients with mood problems and intense sugar cravings take that next step in improvement when their dysbiosis and candida overgrowth are resolved.

Anxiety, agitation, panic attacks, depression, and mood swings are common psychological symptoms (Crook 1997; Jackson et al. 1999) of candida overgrowth. Interestingly, Dr. Leo Galland (1985) reported impaired fatty acid metabolism and low levels of zinc and vitamin B_6 in his patients with candida overgrowth—all nutrients that are vital for mental health and have a bearing on anxiety. Other symptoms include those listed in the candida section of the questionnaire earlier in the chapter, as well as environmental sensitivities, feeling worse on damp or muggy days, insomnia, low blood sugar, PMS, endometriosis, ringing in the ears, headaches, and sensitivities to strong chemical smells (Crook 1997; Lipski 2004).

Testing for Bacterial Imbalance, Parasites, and Candida Overgrowth

The GI Effects Complete Profile, a stool test available from Metametrix (and other stool tests by various labs) can assess for dysbiosis. This test also indicates which medications and natural agents will be effective against your strain of candida or harmful bacteria. Other tests that may be helpful include blood tests for candida antibodies or a white blood cell count. White blood cell levels that are either high (indicating an acute infection) or low (indicating a chronic infection) may indicate a problem when leukocytes, monocytes, or eosinophils (types of white blood cells) are also out of range.

If you don't have access to testing or testing doesn't show candida (as it often doesn't), use the symptoms in the previous questionnaire to assess how you're doing. A big clue that candida may be present is sugar and carbohydrate cravings that are out of control even when taking the amino acids recommended in chapter 6.

Controlling Candida and Increasing Beneficial Bacteria

Controlling candida overgrowth typically requires combining a dietary approach with taking prebiotics, probiotics, and antifungals. There are many wonderful books on the dietary approaches to controlling candida. I encourage you to consult a few and follow their recommendations. In summary, you need to avoid sugar, bread, foods and beverages containing yeast, and possibly even fruit. I really like the simplicity of *Beat Candida Through Diet*, by Gill Jacobs (1997), which discusses the following star foods for candida, including foods that help correct bacterial imbalances, as this will create an environment less favorable to candida:

- Garlic is antifungal, antibacterial, and antiviral, and it helps eliminate toxins. It kills candida and harmful bacteria, increases vitamin absorption, and stimulates production of digestive enzymes. Raw garlic has more of these beneficial properties, but cooked garlic is great too. If you take it in supplement form, buy a freeze-dried product, as this process helps it retain more of its healing properties.

- Onions are anti-inflammatory, antibacterial, and anti-viral, and they help remove parasites. They're also full of antioxidants and are well-known for their many medicinal properties, including helping stave off cancer (Wood 1999).

- Daikon helps maintain a healthy balance of beneficial bacteria.

- Lemons are antibacterial and useful for killing fungi in the mouth and throat.

- Olive oil contains oleic acid, a monounsaturated fat that helps prevent candida overgrowth.

- Raw, unfiltered cider vinegar is rich in potassium and antiseptic and alkalizing, which helps create a good environment for beneficial bacteria.

- Fermented foods and beverages, such as yogurt and sauerkraut, promote good bacterial balance.

The following supplements can be highly effective against candida, but be forewarned: because they can cause a rapid die-off, you could feel worse for a while before you feel better:

- Probiotics are concentrated supplemental forms of the beneficial bacteria that are often depleted in those with candida overgrowth. They increase beneficial bacteria in the gut, helping them crowd out the harmful bacteria. They've also been shown to reduce anxiety and depression (Rao et al. 2009). Look for refrigerated probiotics with lactobacillus, bifidobacteria, and other strains.

- Prebiotics are nondigestible foods, such as soluble fiber, that stimulate the growth of beneficial bacteria in the digestive system. In a study of patients with irritable bowel syndrome (Silk et al. 2009), prebiotics increased bifidobacteria, reduced anxiety and depression, changed stool consistency, and resulted in less bloating. Some examples of prebiotics are psyllium, oat bran, oligofructose, inulin, beta-glucans, and arabinogalactan. All are available in supplement form.

- Oregano oil, grapefruit seed extract, berberine, and caprylic acid are all natural antifungal agents and may be effective for candida. As mentioned, Metametrix's GI Effects Complete Profile will indicate which agents may be effective for your strain of candida.

In an editorial in the *Townsend Letter*, Dr. Alan Gaby (2004) writes in support of this type of approach for vaginal yeast infections, advocating it as a simple, safe, affordable, and effective treatment for chronic yeast infections. He says that despite the fact that there aren't randomized clinical trials supporting this, natural health practitioners have more successful outcomes with these approaches than with medications. I suggest the natural approach first (diet, prebiotics, probiotics, and natural antifungals). If this doesn't work, you may need to work with your doctor and get a prescription for an antifungal medication.

Foods and Nutrients for Healing a Damaged Digestive System

The lining of the intestines can be damaged by food sensitivities, alcohol, medications, and dysbiosis. Once the causative factors are resolved, the gut can start to heal in as little as a week or two, although it can take four to six months for gluten-induced intestinal damage to heal (Braly and Hoggan 2002). The following foods and nutrients are very healing for the digestive system:

- Homemade bone broths (see chapter 1 for a recipe) contain choline, gelatin, and the amino acid proline, nutrients that improve digestion and are very healing to the cells of the digestive tract (Daniel 2003).

- Olive oil is anti-inflammatory and rich in antioxidants and supports the gallbladder (Alarcón de la Lastra et al. 2001).

- Butter contains butyric acid, which is healing for the intestines (Jacobs 1997; Hamer et al. 2008).

- Coconut oil contains lauric acid, which is antibacterial, antiviral, and antifungal (Amarasiri and Dissanayake 2006).

- The amino acid glutamine is the main source of fuel for the small intestine and supports gastrointestinal healing (Miller 1999). It also helps eliminate sugar cravings and maintain blood sugar control (see chapter 2).

- Aloe vera protects and heals the digestive system and has antifungal and anti-inflammatory properties.

Liver or Gallbladder Problems

The liver is the body's main detoxification organ, and supporting it with a two- or three-week seasonal detoxification at least twice a year helps offset the burden of a less-than-ideal diet, caffeine, alcohol, food sensitivities, toxins, dysbiosis, and hormonal imbalances (all of which play a role in anxiety). For a seasonal detoxification program, follow the diet 3 food guidelines in chapter 1, drink plenty of water, avoid gluten and dairy, and use a rice-based product as a source of protein. Here are some additional guidelines:

- Do sauna sessions or Bikram yoga classes to sweat away toxins.

- Use a rebounder or mini trampoline to get your lymphatic system working effectively—important because the lymph carries waste products from the cells.

- Use a dry skin brush before you bathe or shower to remove dead skin cells and enhance elimination of toxins through the skin.

- Use milk thistle, dandelion, and artichoke supplements to further support detoxification.

- Use ox bile and beet supplements to support the gallbladder, which stores bile, needed for fat digestion. The amino acid taurine, which is very calming, also provides liver and gallbladder support.

How Quickly You Can Expect Improvements

Timelines for symptom resolution vary depending on what digestive issues you have. If low stomach acid or pancreatic enzymes are the problem, following the eating guidelines in this chapter and adding hydrochloric acid and digestive enzymes should lead to improvement in a week or two. Balancing bacteria by adding probiotics and fermented foods can be effective within a month, assuming you have sufficient digestive enzymes. Candida can take three months (and often longer) to resolve, especially if mercury toxicity is also an issue (see chapter 8 for more on mercury). Once any damaging agent has been removed (gluten, candida, and so on), nourishing foods and nutrients will aid digestion and start to heal the gut within a few weeks. All of this is based on my experience and time frames may differ from person to person, so it really depends on you and your overall situation.

CHAPTER 6

Balance Brain Chemistry with Amino Acids

This chapter covers the targeted use of individual amino acid supplements for balancing brain chemistry to alleviate anxiety, fear, worry, panic attacks, and feeling stressed or overwhelmed. Supplementing with specific amino acids can also be helpful in addressing other problems that contribute to or exacerbate anxiety, such as sugar cravings and addictions. In addition, supplemental amino acids can help with depression and insomnia, which often co-occur with anxiety. When you balance your brain chemistry, not only will you alleviate symptoms of anxiety, but you'll also have a great mood, eliminate cravings, sleep well, and have good energy and mental focus.

What I mean when I say that "brain chemistry" affects our mood has to do with very specific brain chemicals called neurotransmitters. Neurotransmitters transmit impulses throughout the central nervous system and have a huge impact on mental health and functioning, as well as a wide array of physiological functions. You can balance your brain chemistry by identifying neurotransmitter deficiencies and then raising their levels with amino acid supplements. Amino acids are needed for making neurotransmitters.

It's important to remember that food is the best source of brain-fueling nutrients. You need to eat a wholesome, balanced diet (and remove any foods you could be sensitive to). Proteins are made up of amino acids, and amino acids (together with vitamin and mineral cofactors) are needed to make neurotransmitters, so it's imperative to eat enough good-quality protein, like meat, chicken, eggs, and fish, as well as dairy products if you tolerate them. Eat good-quality protein regularly and make sure you're digesting your protein well (see chapter 5, on digestion). It's also important to make any needed lifestyle changes (chapter 8), since stress affects your brain chemistry. However, sometimes diet and lifestyle aren't enough, and key neurotransmitters remain deficient. Supplements are often the most effective way to deal with this in the short term and in times of stress. Certain amino acids are very effective for specific mood problems and balancing brain chemistry. The key is to use them in a targeted and individualized way, based on your specific symptoms.

Each of the following sections on specific neurotransmitters contains a questionnaire that will help you determine whether you might have a deficiency. Don't be surprised if you appear to have low levels of several neurotransmitters; this is common.

These questionnaires are reprinted from *The Mood Cure* (2004) with permission of Viking Penguin. They do contain a few of my own modifications based on my experience with working with many clients. There is no way to cover, in one chapter, the depth of information in *The Mood Cure* and I encourage you to use this wonderful book, too.

The neurotransmitters we'll look at in this chapter are GABA (gamma-aminobutyric acid), serotonin, catecholamines, and endorphins. GABA plays a major role in anxiety, and serotonin plays a role in at least some types of anxiety (Hoehn-Saric 1982; Nutt 2001). Other neurotransmitters appear to play a lesser role when it comes to anxiety (Hoehn-Saric 1982). I include catecholamines and endorphins even though low levels of these don't appear to be linked to symptoms of anxiety because deficiencies are related to depression, which often occurs with anxiety. You may relate to low catecholamines if you can't live without your coffee (see chapter 3). In addition, all four types of neurotransmitters can be involved in sugar cravings (Ross 2011), and as you learned in chapter 2, sugar and blood sugar swings can play a role in anxiety. If you tried to follow all of the recommendations in chapter 2 but discovered that you're addicted to sugar and cannot give it up, supplemental amino acids can make a world of difference. They can also help with addictions to other refined carbs, drugs, alcohol, and even addictive behaviors, such as gambling (Blum et al. 2000). Low blood sugar could be considered a fifth brain chemistry imbalance with a bearing on anxiety, but I won't discuss it here because this is covered in detail in chapter 2, as is use of the amino acid glutamine to help balance blood sugar.

Before you get started on reading about the individual neurotransmitters and supplementing with amino acids, there's one important caveat. If you appear to have low levels of multiple neurotransmitters, I suggest you begin by taking amino acid supplements to address just one, then gradually add in other amino acids. This way you'll be able to easily assess the improvements. I suggest starting with the deficiency that seems most likely or most problematic for you. Some of my clients find that they have more symptoms of low GABA, while for others alleviating symptoms of low serotonin has the biggest draw. When I'm working with clients I often recommend that they start with more than one amino acid, so if you feel comfortable with this approach, it's an option too.

The great thing about supplementing with amino acids is that you'll get immediate feedback: positive effects, adverse effects, or no changes at all. This allows you to adjust your supplementation until you find the right combination for your unique biochemical needs.

GABA

GABA is the most important calming neurotransmitter and is also an amino acid. Low levels of GABA are associated with anxiety, agitation, stress, and poor sleep (Lydiard 2003; Braverman 2003). If you have sufficient GABA, you'll feel relaxed and stress free. You won't have anxiety or panic attacks, and you won't eat sugary foods (or other starchy foods) in an effort to calm down.

Although there is much clinical evidence that taking supplemental GABA orally can help with anxiety (for example, Ross 2004; Mathews-Larson 2001), there are theories, supported by a few studies, that GABA taken orally doesn't cross the blood-brain barrier and enter into the brain in amounts substantial enough to have a calming effect (Braverman 2003). However, I have seen such dramatic results with GABA, and with so many clients, that I am a firm believer in oral GABA. And there is some evidence to support the effectiveness of a specific formulation of GABA. For example, an unpublished blind study found that 200 mg of PharmaGABA helped people with acrophobia (fear of heights) traverse a suspension bridge that spanned a canyon 150 feet deep (Head and Kelly 2009). That said, I use "regular" GABA with my clients and find it to be extremely effective.

Low GABA Questionnaire

This questionnaire will help you identify whether you may have low levels of GABA. Check off any of the symptoms below that apply to you:

☐ Anxiety and feeling overwhelmed or stressed

☐ Panic attacks

☐ Unable to relax or loosen up

☐ Stiff or tense muscles

☐ Feeling stressed and burned-out

☐ Craving carbs, alcohol, or drugs for relaxation and calming

If you checked off three or more symptoms, the next section may help you improve these symptoms. Worry and anxiety can be a result of low GABA and also low serotonin, so you may check off anxiety in both questionnaires.

Steps to Raise GABA Levels

If you have many of the symptoms of low GABA, you may be amazed at how effective GABA supplementation can be. Within a few minutes of taking a sublingual supplement containing 125 mg of GABA, you'll probably feel more relaxed both mentally and physically.

Take GABA between meals, and be sure to follow the precautions for supplementing with amino acids later in the chapter. Avoid starting with a dose of 750 mg or higher; this is too much for most people. Here are some specific dosages and combinations you might try (to be clear, only use one of these regimens at a time):

- A sublingual supplement containing 125 mg of GABA and 25 mg of tyrosine (for example, GABA Calm, made by Source Naturals): 1 to 2 three times a day or during stressful times (taken between meals).

- 250 to 500 mg of GABA: 1 to 2 at bedtime to help with sleep, or earlier if needed during times of stress (taken between meals)

- Various combination products containing GABA, taurine, and glycine (such as GABA Relaxer, made by Country Life)

In addition to taking supplements, or possibly instead of taking them, try yoga, which has been shown to raise GABA levels (Streeter et al. 2007). It's also important to do whatever you can to reduce stress. In addition to yoga, try tai chi, meditation, taking walks outdoors in a peaceful environment, or taking a vacation.

Serotonin

The neurotransmitter serotonin is the brain's natural "happy, feel-good" chemical. If you have sufficient serotonin, you'll feel calm, easygoing, relaxed, positive, confident, and flexible. You won't have afternoon and evening carb cravings, and you'll sleep well.

While most research on serotonin and its precursors, tryptophan and 5-HTP (5-hydroxytryptophan), has focused on depression, there is evidence that low serotonin is involved in anxiety disorders (Birdsall 1998). Serotonin levels also affect sleep, anger, PMS, carbohydrate cravings, addictive behaviors, and tolerance of heat and pain (ibid.).

Supplements of 5-HTP, the intermediate between tryptophan and serotonin, are obtained from the seeds of the plant *Griffonia simplicifolia.* Unlike other amino acid supplements, 5-HTP can be taken with meals. It increases serotonin levels and is effective for relieving anxiety (ibid.). In particular, it can be helpful with panic attacks (Maron et al. 2004; Lake 2007), agoraphobia (Kahn et al. 1987), and generalized anxiety (Lake 2007). It's also effective for depression, binge eating, carbohydrate cravings, headaches, sleep problems, and fibromyalgia (Birsdall 1998; Ross 2004).

Tryptophan, which first converts to 5-HTP and then to serotonin, has benefits similar to those of 5-HTP (Lehnert and Wurtman 1993; Ross 2004), but there's more research on how 5-HTP affects anxiety. In one study (Zang 1991), 58 percent of patients with generalized anxiety who took 3 grams of tryptophan daily experienced significantly less anxiety. A more recent study (Hudson, Hudson, and MacKenzie 2007) suggests that a functional food rich in tryptophan, made primarily of pumpkin seeds, could be an effective treatment for social anxiety. An hour after eating this functional food, subjects were less anxious when asked to speak in front of others.

Low Serotonin Questionnaire

This questionnaire will help you identify whether you may have low levels of serotonin. Check off any of the symptoms below that apply to you:

☐ Anxiety

☐ Panic attacks or phobias

☐ Feeling worried or fearful

☐ Obsessive thoughts or behaviors

☐ Perfectionism or being overly controlling

☐ Irritability

☐ Anxiety that's worse in winter

☐ Winter blues or seasonal affective disorder

☐ Negativity or depression

☐ Suicidal thoughts

☐ Excessive self-criticism

☐ Low self-esteem and poor self-confidence

☐ PMS or menopausal mood swings

☐ Sensitivity to hot weather

☐ Hyperactivity

☐ Anger or rage

☐ Digestive issues

☐ Fibromyalgia, temporomandibular joint syndrome (TMJ), or other pain syndromes

☐ Difficulty getting to sleep before 10 p.m.

☐ Insomnia or disturbed sleep

☐ Afternoon or evening cravings for carbs, alcohol, or drugs

If you checked off six or more symptoms, the next section may help you improve these symptoms. Worry and anxiety can be a result of low GABA and also low serotonin, so you may check off anxiety in both questionnaires. But if you have other symptoms of low serotonin and low GABA, you may need to address both deficiencies.

Steps to Raise Serotonin Levels

If you have many of the symptoms of low serotonin and feel anxious and negative, you may notice a calmness and elevation in mood after supplementing with tryptophan or 5-HTP. You might even start to smile and joke.

You may experience greater benefits with tryptophan or with 5-HTP (Ross 2004), so try one and then the other and use whichever form works best for you. 5-HTP sometimes causes mild nausea, but this usually abates after a few days. You could switch to tryptophan instead. If you have severe insomnia or often feel "tired but wired," take tryptophan rather than 5-HTP, since 5-HTP can raise levels of the stress hormone cortisol and thereby disrupt sleep. If you don't know if you have high cortisol, I suggest starting with tryptophan, even though it's more expensive. One word of caution: If you're currently taking a selective serotonin reuptake inhibitor (SSRI) or monoamine oxidase inhibitor (MAOI), don't take either 5-HTP or tryptophan unless you're working with a knowledgeable practitioner. And be sure to read and understand the amino acid precautions and information on serotonin syndrome below.

If you decide that supplementing with tryptophan or 5-HTP may be helpful for you, here are specific dosages you might try (to be clear, only use one of these regimens at a time):

- 500 to 1,500 mg of tryptophan: twice a day, midafternoon and at bedtime (taken between meals)

- 50 to 150 mg of 5-HTP: twice a day, midafternoon and at bedtime (can be taken with food)

- For symptoms that occur earlier in the day, 50 to 150 mg of 5-HTP on waking and midmorning, and 500 to 1,500 mg of tryptophan midafternoon and at bedtime

Moderate exercise raises serotonin levels and relieves anxiety (Petruzzello et al. 1991), specifically OCD and phobias (Tkachuk and Martin 1999). Getting regular exercise, if you aren't already doing so, is an important lifestyle change to make (see chapter 8 for more on exercise). Exercise also raises levels of endorphins and therefore can help with sadness and comfort eating. But too much exercise can raise anxiety-producing cortisol.

Sunshine and light therapy will also raise serotonin levels. There's evidence of seasonality in anxiety and panic attacks, as there is with seasonal affective disorder (SAD). Light therapy, such as a full-spectrum lamp (3,000-10,000 lux), during the winter months may be effective for alleviating symptoms if you tend to get the winter blues or feel more anxious when it's less sunny (Marriott, Greenwood, and Armstrong 1994). It's also possible that remedying any deficiency of vitamin D could improve seasonal anxiety and depression (Lansdowne and Provost 1998).

Catecholamines

Catecholamines are hormones produced by the brain and adrenal glands in response to stress. The most abundant catecholamines are epinephrine (adrenaline), norepinephrine (noradrenaline), and dopamine. If you have sufficient catecholamines, you'll feel energized, upbeat, alert, and focused, and you won't be craving a quick pick-me-up, like an afternoon soda or candy. Low levels of catecholamines can lead to the kind of depression that's a curl-up-in-bed feeling, where you have very low motivation and don't want to see anyone.

Because catecholamines are produced and utilized in the fight-or-flight response, stress depletes them. Supplementing with their precursor, the amino acid tyrosine, can improve mood and memory and improve your ability to tolerate stressful situations (Banderet and Lieberman 1989). It can also help eliminate sugar, caffeine, and chocolate cravings and other addictive behaviors (Blum et al. 2000).

Low Catecholamines Questionnaire

This questionnaire will help you identify whether you may have low levels of catecholamines. Check off any of the following symptoms that apply to you:

- ☐ Depression with apathy
- ☐ Easily bored
- ☐ Lack of energy
- ☐ Lack of focus
- ☐ Lack of drive and low motivation
- ☐ Attention deficit disorder

☐ Procrastination and indecisiveness

☐ Craving carbs, alcohol, caffeine, or drugs for energy

If you checked off three or more items, the section below may help you improve these symptoms.

Steps to Raise Catecholamine Levels

If you have many of the symptoms of low catecholamines and you feel fatigued or unfocused, you may notice an immediate increase in energy and focus after taking supplemental tyrosine.

Try taking 500 to 1,500 mg of tyrosine one to three times a day, before breakfast, midmorning, and midafternoon. Take tyrosine between meals, and don't take it later than 3:00 p.m. if you have insomnia. Tyrosine is particularly helpful if you need coffee to get going in the morning (and as you learned in chapter 3, quitting coffee can help alleviate your anxiety). One caveat with tyrosine: there's a chance that it could make your anxiety worse. If it does, you may need to supplement with GABA, 5-HTP, or tryptophan to increase your levels of calming neurotransmitters before you start taking tyrosine.

Omega-3s and vitamin D also play a role in catecholamine production (Ross 2004), so have your fatty acid and vitamin D levels checked. Also have your levels of thyroid and adrenal hormones checked, since low levels of catecholamines may indicate dysfunction in either or both of these endocrine glands (see chapter 8). And be aware that all of these factors can also contribute to depression and lethargy.

Endorphins

Endorphins are neurotransmitters that reduce physical and emotional pain. You may be familiar with the term "runner's high," which refers to the effects of endorphins that are released at a certain level of exertion. If you have sufficient endorphins, you'll feel pleasure and joy, similar to the feeling you get when someone gives you a big hug. You also won't be drawn to eating sweet or fatty foods to comfort yourself.

The amino acid D-phenylalanine inhibits the enzyme that breaks down endorphins (Ross 2004), so supplementing with it, as either D-phenylalanine (DPA) or DL-phenylalanine (DLPA), will help raise endorphin levels and resolve symptoms of low endorphins. DPA is more potent for raising endorphins and is one of my favorite supplements. DLPA is an option if you also have symptoms of low catecholamines, as some of it will be converted to tyrosine. However, it has less of an impact on raising endorphins for some people.

Low Endorphins Questionnaire

This questionnaire will help you identify whether you may have low levels of endorphins. Check off any of the following symptoms that apply to you:

- ☐ Sensitivity to emotional pain

- ☐ Sensitivity to physical pain

- ☐ Crying or tearing up easily

- ☐ Eating to soothe your mood, or comfort eating

- ☐ Really, really *loving* certain foods, behaviors, drugs, or alcohol

- ☐ Craving a reward or numbing treat

If you checked off more than three items, the section below will help you improve these symptoms.

Steps to Raise Endorphin Levels

When you have low endorphins, you may find that you really love certain foods and may eat these foods as a way of comforting yourself. I often hear clients say things like, "Oh, I just *love* chocolate," or "I *love* bread so much," with that special smile where their eyes light up. Clients may be almost tearful when they consider the idea of giving up these foods. But shortly after taking some DPA (or DLPA), they're generally able to say, "Oh, I could just take it or leave it right now," and they're quite surprised that it works that effectively and that quickly. Here are some specific dosages and combinations you might try, all taken between meals (to be clear, only use one of these regimens at a time):

- 500 to 1,500 mg DPA: three times a day, before breakfast, midmorning, and midafternoon. You may also need some after dinner.

- 500 to 1,500 mg DLPA: three times a day, before breakfast, midmorning, and midafternoon. DLPA may be useful if you have low energy and also tend to engage in comfort eating. If you have insomnia, avoid DLPA altogether or don't take it after 3:00 p.m.

If supplementing with DPA or DLPA, be sure to eat sufficient good-quality protein and take a free-form amino acid blend with all nine essential amino acids, including tryptophan, to support your body's production of endorphins. Free-form amino acids don't require digestion and are very easily absorbed.

Also, consider whether sensitivity to gluten or dairy may be an issue (covered in chapter 4), as these foods can produce a drug-like effect, similar to an endorphin high, that can be addicting. Exercise, meditation, and acupuncture can all help raise endorphin levels. Interestingly, acts of generosity, such as doing nice things for others, can also raise endorphin levels. So can deep breathing, good memories, a hug, being out in nature, being in love, or a massage. Cranial electrical stimulation, an FDA-approved approach for treating depression, pain, and insomnia, also raises levels of both endorphins and serotonin.

■ My Story

When I was in my late thirties, I had a very stressful computer job. I worked long hours, and as the months went on, my problem with anxiety was getting worse and worse, yet there was nothing concrete that I could attribute my anxiety to. I often woke up in the night and early hours with a pounding heart and a sense of impending doom that I found difficult to explain. Then I had three panic attacks over a three-week period. Within a week of starting to take two GABA Calm supplements twice a day, my anxiety was significantly reduced. I also started taking two GABA Relaxer supplements at bedtime, which further reduced my nighttime anxiety and helped me feel calmer and more relaxed. I've never had another panic attack since.

This is my story with GABA. I also have pyroluria and gluten sensitivity, and back then I suffered from adrenal fatigue and low progesterone. The GABA helped right away while I started to investigate and address my other issues.

You may need more than one amino acid. See other stories in other chapters and appendix 1 for Sue's story. She benefited from 5-HTP, GABA, and DPA.

Testing for Levels of Amino Acids

The symptom questionnaire developed by Julia Ross, covered extensively in *The Mood Cure* (2004) and used at her Recovery Systems Clinic for over twenty years, is a very effective method of assessing for brain chemistry imbalances. It has been used successfully in many other settings and clinics. Many health practitioners have completed the amino acid training offered by Julia Ross and use her questionnaire and amino acid protocols.

One of the reasons Julia Ross's approach is so effective is because, based on results of the questionnaires, her nutritionists have clients take the indicated amino acids on a trial basis right away—then and there in the clinic. I do the same with all my clients. Because the effects of amino acids can be felt within a few minutes to a few days, it's easy to confirm whether you do in fact have a deficiency in a certain area and whether you'll benefit from supplementing with the associated amino acid.

For serotonin and the catecholamines, a platelet test (offered by Health Diagnostics and Research Institute) is another option for assessing levels. This is an especially good idea if you suffer from severe depression and anxiety, or during pregnancy and breastfeeding. Platelet testing appears to be more closely correlated with levels of these neurotransmitters in the cerebrospinal fluid than other types of tests, such as urinary neurotransmitter testing. I don't have clinical experience with urinary neurotransmitter testing, but Julia Ross (2006) has found it to be unreliable, despite its popularity. Plasma testing of neurotransmitters also appears to be less reliable than platelet testing but more reliable than urine testing.

Drug of Choice

Sometimes it's difficult to figure out why you're drawn to a particular food, substance, or behavior and which part of your brain chemistry it's affecting, and you may not associate cravings with mood issues. This section provides additional guidance on figuring out why you may crave certain things. Your drug of choice is whatever makes you feel good or "normal." It could be candy, chocolate, starchy foods like bread, cigarettes, alcohol, marijuana, a prescription medication like Prozac, street drugs, or even shopping or exercise. Cravings for these substances (or behaviors) typically indicate a brain chemistry imbalance, so it's very helpful to identify how the substances you crave affect you. This will help you determine which amino acids you might supplement to address the imbalance. For example, tobacco may be calming for one person but energizing for another, or chocolate may be calming for some people and comforting for others. Certain prescription medications also offer clues. If you have many symptoms of low serotonin and have found that prescription SSRIs help, it's likely that low serotonin is an issue.

Taking chocolate as an example, here's what I suggest: Before you eat some chocolate, think about why you want it. Is it because you're sad or tired or anxious? Or do you feel that you deserve a reward or feel irritable and shaky? Then, once you've eaten it, think about how it made you feel. Finally, use the following chart to help you determine what brain chemistry imbalance may be affecting you.

How you feel before	How you feel after	Brain chemistry imbalance	Amino acid to supplement
Anxious or stressed	Calm or relaxed	Low GABA	GABA
Depressed or anxious	Happy or content	Low serotonin	Tryptophan or 5-HTP
Tired or unfocused	Energetic, alert, or focused	Low catecholamines	Tyrosine
Wanting a reward or feeling sad	Rewarded or comforted	Low endorphins	DPA, DLPA
Irritable and shaky	Grounded or stable	Low blood sugar	Glutamine (see chapter 2)

Guidelines for Supplementing with Amino Acids

Use the questionnaires in this chapter to assess any neurotransmitter imbalances carefully, and take only the amino acids that you need. Take amino acids thirty minutes before or sixty minutes after a meal containing protein, with the exception of 5-HTP, which can be taken with meals. You'll experience the benefits more quickly if you take a sublingual form or chew the supplement. You can just chew the gelatin capsule. DPA has a pleasant taste, but with the other amino acids, chewing them isn't the most pleasant experience. Sublingual GABA is particularly effective and the flavor is pleasant.

People's responses to amino acids vary. You may notice nothing, you may experience relief from symptoms, or you may have an adverse effect, such as a headache or light-headed feeling. With all amino acids (and any other supplements, for that matter), if you experience any adverse effects, stop taking them immediately. If adverse effects of supplemental amino acids are uncomfortable, taking 1,000 mg of vitamin C is an effective short-term antidote.

Always respect the reverse effect of nutrients: Excesses can often be problematic, and may even have the same effect as a deficiency. Start with the lowest recommended dose of amino acids and increase from there as needed, keeping in mind that you may need an even lower dose, especially if you're very sensitive to supplements. Some of my very sensitive clients take less than one-fifth the lowest recommended dose. If you're similar, you can open a capsule to take a smaller portion.

Amino acids typically aren't needed long term if you eat a whole foods diet and get enough protein. Three to six months of supplementation is generally sufficient to resolve deficiencies. About a month after your symptoms have resolved, gradually taper your dose. Once you haven't been taking the amino acid for about three months, use the questionnaires in this chapter to assess whether you still have a deficiency. Also be aware that you may need to supplement with certain amino acids during winter if your anxiety or depression reappears or worsens. The same is true for times of high or ongoing stress. Some people need amino acids for as long as a year but rarely longer.

Amino Acid Precautions

There are some precautions to be aware of when taking supplemental amino acids. These are reprinted from *The Mood Cure* (2004) with permission of Viking Penguin. Consult a knowledgeable practitioner before taking *any* supplemental amino acids if any of the following statements applies to you:

- You react to supplements, foods, or medications with unusual or uncomfortable symptoms.

- You have a serious physical illness, particularly cancer.

- You have severe liver or kidney problems.

- You have an ulcer (amino acids are slightly acidic).

- You have schizophrenia or another mental illness, such as bipolar disorder.

- You are pregnant or nursing.

- You are taking any medications for mood problems, particularly MAOIs or more than one SSRI.

Also, please be aware of the following precautions in regard to specific amino acids and consult with a knowledgeable practitioner if in doubt.

Do you have?	If yes, do not take these
Overactive thyroid or Grave's disease	Tyrosine, DLPA
Phenylketonuria (PKU)	Tyrosine, DLPA
Melanoma	Tyrosine, DLPA
High blood pressure	Tyrosine, DLPA
Migraine headaches	Tyrosine, DLPA
Low blood pressure	GABA or taurine
Asthma	Tryptophan or melatonin
Severe depression	Melatonin
Bipolar disorder	Tyrosine, DLPA, or glutamine

Amino Acids and SSRIs

If you're currently taking a selective serotonin reuptake inhibitor (SSRI) or monoamine oxidase inhibitor (MAOI), don't take either 5-HTP or tryptophan unless you're working with a knowledgeable practitioner. Taking 5-HTP or tryptophan with either of these classes of antidepressants may cause serotonin syndrome (Birdsall 1998), an adverse reaction characterized by agitation, confusion, rapid heart rate, and blood pressure fluctuations. If you experience these symptoms, stop taking 5-HTP or tryptophan immediately. When I have clients who are taking a single SSRI who might also benefit from tryptophan or 5-HTP, I have them take the amino acid six hours apart from their medications—after obtaining approval from their doctors and with their doctors monitoring for adverse reactions. Please do the same. I also recommend the chapter on antidepressants and amino acids in *The Mood Cure* (2004).

How Quickly You Can Expect Improvements

If you have a brain chemistry imbalance and take the needed amino acid, you can expect noticeable improvements within a few minutes, and often dramatic improvements within a day. It is very easy to remember to take the amino acids you need, because you'll notice an immediate turn for the worse if you miss a dose. It typically isn't necessary to supplement with specific amino acids for more than three to six months if you eat a whole foods diet and get enough protein.

CHAPTER 7

Address Pyroluria or Low Levels of Zinc and Vitamin B$_6$

Low levels of the mineral zinc and vitamin B$_6$ are frequently associated with a type of anxiety characterized by social anxiety, avoidance of crowds, a feeling of inner tension, and bouts of depression. People with this problem experience varying degrees of anxiety or fear, often starting in childhood, but they usually manage to cover it up. They tend to build their lives around one person, become more of a loner over time, have difficulty handling stress or change, and have heightened anxiety symptoms when under more stress.

This constellation of symptoms is often the result of a genetic condition called *pyroluria*, also known as high mauve, pyrrole disorder, pyrroluria, pyrolleuria, malvaria, and elevated kryptopyrroles. For simplicity I use the term "pyroluria" in this chapter and elsewhere in the book.

In *Nutrition and Mental Illness* (1987), Carl Pfeiffer describes pyroluria as faulty synthesis of heme (a component of hemoglobin, in the blood), resulting in elevated levels of kryptopyrroles (KP) or by-products of hemoglobin synthesis that have no known role in the body. To get quite technical, it turns out that what's elevated is actually levels of another molecule: hydroxyhemopyrrolin-2-one (HPL; McGinnis et al. 2008a, 2008b). This molecule attaches to zinc and vitamin B_6 in the body, which are then excreted in greater amounts than normal in the urine, resulting in deficiencies. Supplementing with zinc and vitamin B_6 improves the many signs and symptoms of pyroluria (ibid.; Mathews-Larson 2001). HPL also inhibits synthesis of heme (McGinnis et al. 2008a, 2008b), explaining why people with pyroluria often also have low levels of iron or ferritin (the body's storage form of iron and the first indicator of decreased iron levels) and need to supplement with iron as well.

Pyroluria Questionnaire

This questionnaire will help you identify whether you might have pyroluria. The physical and emotional symptoms below are caused by deficiencies of vitamin B_6 and zinc. When you experience high levels of stress, vitamin B_6 and zinc will be further depleted, so you may notice worsening symptoms and more anxiety.

Based on my review of questionnaires and results of pyroluria tests for hundreds of clients, I've grouped the most common or classic signs and symptoms first. I've also labeled the symptoms that could be directly related to low levels of vitamin B_6 or zinc so you can individualize your supplements and dosages. Symptoms without these designations are due to a deficiency of both vitamin B_6 and zinc. Check off any of the following signs or symptoms that apply to you:

Most Common Signs and Symptoms

- ☐ Being anxious, shy, or fearful, or experiencing inner tension since childhood, but hiding these feelings from others

- ☐ Having bouts of depression or nervous exhaustion

- ☐ Poor dream recall, stressful or bizarre dreams, or nightmares (low vitamin B_6)

☐ Excessive reactions to tranquilizers, barbiturates, alcohol, or other drugs, in which a little produces a powerful response (low vitamin B_6)

☐ Preferring not to eat breakfast, experiencing light nausea in the morning, or being prone to motion sickness (low vitamin B_6)

☐ White spots or flecks on the fingernails, or opaquely white or paper-thin nails (low zinc)

☐ Liquid zinc sulfate having a mild taste or tasting like water (low zinc)

☐ Poor appetite or having a poor sense of smell or taste (low zinc)

☐ Joints popping, cracking, or aching; pain or discomfort between the shoulder blades; or cartilage problems (low zinc)

☐ Pale or fair skin or being the palest in the family, or sunburning easily, now or when younger

☐ Disliking protein or having ever been a vegetarian or vegan

☐ Being sensitive to bright sunlight or noise

☐ Upper abdominal pain on your left side under the ribs or, as a child, having a stitch in your side as you ran

☐ Frequent fatigue

☐ Being prone to iron anemia or low ferritin levels

☐ Tending to have cold hands or feet

☐ Having frequent colds or infections, or unexplained chills or fever

☐ Reaching puberty later than normal or having irregular menstruation or PMS

☐ Having allergies, adrenal issues, or problems with sugar metabolism

☐ Having gluten sensitivity

☐ Neurotransmitter imbalances, especially low serotonin

☐ For women, belonging to an all-girl family or having look-alike sisters

☐ For men, having a mother from an all-girl family or a mother with look-alike sisters, or all the females in the mother's family bearing a strong resemblance to each other

☐ Avoiding stress because it upsets your emotional balance

☐ Tending to become dependent on one person whom you build your life around

☐ Preferring the company of one or two close friends rather than a gathering of friends; becoming more of a loner as you age

☐ Feeling uncomfortable with strangers

☐ Being bothered by being seated in the middle of the room in a restaurant

☐ Being easily upset by criticism

Less Common Signs and Symptoms

☐ Stretch marks or poor wound healing (low zinc)

☐ Crowded upper front teeth, many cavities, or inflamed gums or wearing braces (low zinc)

☐ Bad breath and body odor (or a sweet, fruity odor), especially when ill or stressed (low zinc)

☐ Being prone to acne, eczema, herpes, or psoriasis

☐ Reduced amount of hair on your head, eyebrows, or eyelashes, or prematurely gray hair

☐ Difficultly recalling past events and people in your life

☐ Focusing internally, on yourself, rather than on the external world

☐ Tending to have morning constipation

☐ Tingling sensations or muscle spasms in your legs or arms

☐ Feeling stressed by changes in your routine, such as traveling or being in new situations

☐ Having a swollen-appearing face when you're under a lot of stress

☐ Cluster headaches or blinding headaches

☐ One or more of the following: a psychiatric disorder, schizophrenia, high or low histamine, alcoholism, learning and behavioral disorders, autism, or Down syndrome

If you check off fifteen or more items, especially the more common ones, it's highly probable that you have pyroluria and will benefit from taking zinc and vitamin B_6 supplements. I encourage you to be tested, but if this isn't possible, or even if you don't have pyroluria, supplementing with zinc and vitamin B_6 may be worthwhile if you have a large number of these symptoms.

This questionnaire is based on my experience working with many clients with pyroluria, along with information from *Depression-Free Naturally* (2001), by Joan Mathews-Larson; *Nutrition and Mental Illness* (1987), by Carl Pfeiffer; and *Natural Healing for Schizophrenia and Other Common Mental Disorders* (2001), by Eva Edelman.

Prevalence of Pyroluria and Co-occurring Disorders

Much of what we know about pyroluria is based on the work of Humphrey Osmond, Abram Hoffer, and Carl Pfeiffer (Pfeiffer et al. 1974). Much of the original work was done with schizophrenic patients in psychiatric hospital settings, but pyroluria has since been found in people with many different disorders and even in those with no diagnosis. Although pyroluria was first identified in the 1960s, the medical and mental health communities have been slow to recognize it, and many mental health practitioners and physicians remain unfamiliar with this condition.

Estimates of the prevalence of pyroluria vary. Joan Mathews-Larson (2001), considered an expert on the subject, reports the prevalence as follows: 11 percent of the healthy population, 40 percent of adults with psychiatric disorders, 25 percent of children with psychiatric disorders, 30 percent of people with schizophrenia, and 40 percent of alcoholics. Abram Hoffer (1995) worked primarily with schizophrenic patients, but he found pyroluria was also present in 25 percent of his nonschizophrenic patients, including adults with anxiety, depression, and alcoholism, and children with learning disorders and behavioral disorders. Pyroluria is also present in about 46 percent of people with autism spectrum disorders and 71 percent of those with Down syndrome (McGinnis et al. 2008a, 2008b). I work primarily with adult women who are anxious, depressed, or both, and have found that at least 80 percent of my clients with moderate to severe anxiety have a large number of pyroluria symptoms.

The typical age of onset is the late teenage years, but it's entirely possible for symptoms of pyroluria to surface earlier, especially if stress is a factor, for example, if a baby has a stressful birth or undergoes surgery or another trauma, or a child loses a best friend, changes schools, or has parents going through a divorce. The symptoms can range from very severe to very mild, depending on the person's biochemistry and how extreme the imbalance is. And as discussed, symptom severity is also greatly affected by stress.

As mentioned, pyroluria is an inherited condition, and it often shows up in families with a history of mental illnesses or addiction. Multiple family members often have pyroluria symptoms. So if you discover you have pyroluria, consider sharing the questionnaire with other family members, particularly your mother, grandmother, sisters, and daughters, as it seems to affect females more than males.

An interesting observation is that pyroluria and gluten sensitivity often co-occur in people with anxiety, depression, autism, alcoholism and other addictions, bipolar disorder, or schizophrenia. So be sure to read the material on gluten sensitivity in chapter 4 carefully; it may be helpful for you. Pyroluria also sometimes occurs along with histamine imbalances and allergies that affect brain function (Pfeiffer et al. 1974), also covered in chapter 4. Adrenal problems (covered in chapter 8) and digestive problems (the topic of chapter 5) also commonly co-occur with pyroluria. Because both zinc and vitamin B_6 are important for neurotransmitter production, if you have pyroluria your levels of serotonin and GABA may also be low (see chapter 6 for more on neurotransmitters). Finally, taking large amounts of vitamin B_6 can deplete levels of magnesium, so be sure to also read the section on magnesium (in chapter 8).

Testing for Pyroluria

The tests described below can determine whether you might have pyroluria and help you assess improvements. You may be able to confirm if you have pyroluria with a urine test. You can do an initial zinc status check with the zinc taste test, and then retest in several weeks to determine whether your zinc levels are improving. To assess changes in vitamin B_6 status, monitor your dream recall or consider organic acids testing. I also recommend fatty acid testing, since many people with pyroluria need specific omega-6 fatty acids, rather than omega-3s.

Pyroluria Urine Test

Historically, Vitamin Diagnostics, a specialty lab now called Health Diagnostics and Research Institute, offered a reliable and a very affordable at-home urine pyroluria test. They plan to start offering it again in 2011. Although a number of other labs offer pyroluria tests, the results, unfortunately, are not as reliable. This may be due in part to the fact that the substance measured, HPL, is fragile and unstable in light.

It's important to stop taking supplemental zinc and vitamin B_6 at least two weeks before collecting urine for the test. If testing indicates that you have pyroluria, you will always need to take supplemental zinc and vitamin B_6, but you can only determine how much by monitoring your zinc and vitamin B_6 status. Once your symptoms abate, you might be fine with what you get from a good multivitamin, or you might need more zinc or vitamin B_6.

Zinc Taste Test

While there is no generally accepted standard for measuring zinc, the zinc taste test can provide some guidance. This uses liquid zinc sulfate, which you can purchase from a nutritionist. Zinc affects your taste buds, so your taste response to holding about 2 tablespoons of zinc sulfate in your mouth for thirty seconds indicates the extent of your zinc deficiency. This is called the zinc taste test or zinc tally.

- Category 1 indicates the greatest need for supplemental zinc. At this level, there is no specific taste or sensation; you may think the solution tastes like water.

- Category 2 indicates a moderate need for zinc. At this level, you won't immediately notice any taste, but after a few seconds you'll detect a slight taste that may seem stale, furry, chalky, or sweet, or have a dry mineral quality.

- Category 3 indicates less of a need for zinc. Almost immediately, you'll notice a definite mildly unpleasant taste that tends to intensify with time.

- Category 4 indicates no need for extra zinc beyond the amount found in a multivitamin, which is about 15 mg. You'll notice a very strong and unpleasant taste right away, and it's unpleasant enough that you'll want to spit it out immediately. In this case, it's okay to spit it out immediately.

Zinc deficiency is very common. The zinc status of most of my anxious clients is category 1 or 2, and for many of my clients who don't have anxiety, it's category 2 or 3.

In my experience, plasma and serum zinc levels don't correlate with the zinc taste test, low zinc symptoms, or pyroluria test results. However low serum levels of alkaline phosphatase, an enzyme, may be an indication of low zinc status (Lord and Bralley 2008). And fatty acid testing, covered below, may also be useful, as certain fatty acid ratios can help to determine whether you're deficient in zinc. I'll discuss zinc supplements and dietary sources of zinc in detail later.

Vitamin B$_6$ Testing

Your dreams and dream recall serve as a good indicator of your need for vitamin B$_6$. You should dream and remember your dreams most nights. They should be pleasant—the kind of dreams where you wake up and want to close your eyes and continue dreaming.

If you don't remember your dreams or if you have disturbing, stressful, or weird dreams or nightmares, you probably need vitamin B$_6$, even if you don't have pyroluria or don't score 15 or more on the questionnaire. Supplementing with vitamin B$_6$ will improve your dream recall and quality (Mathews-Larson 2001; McGinnis et al. 2008a, 2008b). Keep taking supplemental vitamin B$_6$ until you start to remember your dreams or you no longer have nightmares.

Organic acids are products of metabolism that can identify nutrient deficiencies, including low levels of vitamin B$_6$, so organic acids testing (available from Metametrix) can be helpful. Xanthurenate and kynurenate are organic acids. Elevated levels of xanthurenate in the urine can indicate an insufficiency of vitamin B$_6$, as can elevated levels of kynurenate, especially when xanthurenate is high (Lord and Bralley 2008). I'll discuss vitamin B$_6$ supplements and dietary sources of vitamin B$_6$ in detail later.

Fatty Acid Testing

These days, fish oil and other omega-3 supplements are highly popular and almost universally touted for their health benefits, especially for depression. Omega-3s are indeed highly beneficial, but if you have pyroluria, you can probably extract the omega-3s eicosapentaenoic acid (EPA) and docosahexaenoic acid (DHA) from foods such as oily fish; walnuts; leafy, green vegetables; and, if grass-fed, red meat. For people with pyroluria who are getting enough omega-3s from food, it's important not to take them as supplements, because this can worsen symptoms if you aren't deficient.

Pyroluria causes changes in fatty acid metabolism (Heleniak and Lamola 1986; McGinnis et al. 2008a, 2008b) that often lead to low levels of the omega-6 fatty acids gamma-linolenic acid (GLA) and arachidonic acid (AA). GLA, found in evening primrose oil and borage oil, is also beneficial for those with pyroluria because it improves zinc absorption (McGinnis et al. 2008a, 2008b). Arachadonic acid is abundant in red meat, eggs, butter, and liver, so be sure to include these foods in your diet if arachidonic acid is low.

Fatty acid testing can also help determine whether you may be deficient in zinc. If the ratio of linoleic acid to dihomo-gamma-linoleic acid (LA:DGLA) is high, you may have a zinc deficiency. This is because zinc is necessary for the action of an enzyme involved in fatty acid conversions (Lord and Bralley 2008). As mentioned, fatty acid tests for those with pyroluria will often show low levels of GLA, as well as low DGLA, and adequate levels of EPA and DHA.

Among my clients with pyroluria, I've seen many test results confirming this need for omega-6s rather than omega-3s. However, a handful did need omega-3s, so the best bet is to test periodically to determine your unique needs, and then supplement as needed. Fatty acid tests are available from Metametrix and Health Diagnostics and Research Institute (formerly Vitamin Diagnostics).

Comprehensive Metabolic Profile

Organic acids and fatty acids are both assessed in the Comprehensive Metabolic Profile (CMP) offered by Metametrix. This panel is particularly helpful because it also assesses for sensitivity to thirty common foods, dybiosis markers, liver function, B vitamin status, antioxidant status, and some neurotransmitters.

■ Samantha's Story

Samantha, a thirty-four-year-old health professional and new mom, ate reasonably well but admitted to being a huge fan of all sweet foods. The only supplement she took was a multivitamin, and even that she didn't take regularly. She had recently started experiencing increasing anxiety and scored over 15 on the pyroluria questionnaire. She described her anxiety like this: "I have a feeling of nervousness I can't explain. I can't put a finger on what's making me nervous. My anxiety is especially worse in social situations and not as bad when I'm at home."

She wasn't willing to do a urine test for pyroluria and wasn't a believer in supplements, but she reluctantly agreed to try taking 30 mg of zinc and 100 mg of vitamin B_6 daily. This was the only change she made, yet she noticed some improvements in her anxiety within a week, and a huge reduction over the next month. Because she wasn't completely convinced the zinc and vitamin B_6 were responsible for the change, she started to be less conscientious about taking them, thinking all was well. Within a week she was starting to feel nervous again.

She started taking the supplements again, and sure enough, her nervousness diminished. After a few more on-off trials, she was finally convinced that she does need these supplements daily, though she has found that when she's less stressed and eats less sugar, she can take less of both supplements.

Zinc, Vitamin B_6, and Fatty Acids for Pyroluria

I've found that everyone who scores 20 or more on the pyroluria questionnaire tests positive for pyroluria, and that those with scores of 15 to 19 often test positive as well. If you score 15 or more, it's likely that you need more zinc and vitamin B_6, whether you have pyroluria or not. However, some of the less common symptoms could be related to other causes: Cold hands and feet could be due to low thyroid. Anemia could be caused by low amounts of iron in the diet. Constipation could be due to poor diet, insufficient fiber, or low thyroid function. And joint aches and pains could be caused by low levels of fatty acids or food sensitivities.

Zinc Supplementation

Some researchers have found that supplementing with 25 to 100 mg of zinc daily (in conjunction with vitamin B$_6$) usually results in dramatic reduction of pyroluria symptoms, and this is a level of supplementation that they deem safe (McGinnis et al. 2008b). There have also been many studies on the importance of zinc for nervous system function and its role in emotional disorders (Prasad 1985; Wallwork 1987).

I suggest starting with 30 mg daily and then increasing to 60 mg. However, if urine testing confirms that you have pyroluria, it's probably safe to initially supplement with 90 mg daily. Whatever amount you take, monitor your zinc levels with the zinc taste test. You should notice that the liquid zinc sulfate starts to taste increasingly worse, though initially it may just seem to change in texture, becoming more dry and chalky. I typically have clients take 30 to 60 mg of zinc a day, and never more than 90 mg. Reduce the amount you take as the zinc sulfate taste gets stronger.

I've found that OptiZinc, a patented form of zinc monomethionine available in some brands, to be very effective for most of my clients. This form of zinc has a reputation for being the most readily used by the body. But since we are all unique, another form, such as zinc picolinate or chelate, may work better for you. Supplementing with zinc can be a challenge; some people don't absorb it very well. I often need to switch the forms clients are taking until we find something that works. If you supplement for one month and change forms and the taste test still doesn't indicate any improvement in zinc status, I suggest that you avoid gluten if you aren't doing so already, as gluten sensitivity can impair mineral absorption.

The recommended dietary allowance (RDA) of zinc is low: just 8 to 12 mg a day for adults. I think this is too low even for the average person. The current guideline for upper tolerable limit is 40 mg a day, so when taking amounts much above 60 mg daily, I suggest working with a holistic practitioner. One of the commonly raised concerns around taking higher doses of zinc is that it can have a negative impact on the zinc-copper balance, resulting in levels of copper that are too low. However, this doesn't tend to happen often, as we typically get plenty of copper from dietary sources. Vegetarian diets tend to be especially high in copper and low in zinc. High copper levels can also be caused by copper in pipes (and therefore drinking water), cooking pots, and IUDs, and by taking oral contraceptives. If you're trying to raise your zinc levels, make sure there isn't any copper in your zinc supplement (there often is). For some of my very anxious clients, even copper in a multivitamin is an issue. There are a few companies currently making multivitamins that are copper free, including Designs for Health.

Zinc is depleted by stress, exercise, and excessive sugar consumption, so you may need to adjust your dosage depending on these factors. Taking too much zinc or taking a form your body doesn't tolerate may result in nausea; for example, some people feel sick on zinc picolinate but don't have a problem with OptiZinc. To help prevent nausea, also take zinc with meals.

Food Sources of Zinc

It's good to try to get more zinc from your diet, but if you have pyroluria, you will also need to supplement with zinc. Here are some of the best food sources:

- The highest concentration of zinc is in oysters, and they contain more zinc when raw.

- Other shellfish, such as mussels, shrimp, and crab, are rich in zinc.

- Red meat, fish, and chicken are good sources of zinc.

- Cheeses such as ricotta, Swiss, and Gouda are relatively high in zinc.

- Zinc is also found in smaller amounts in whole grains, beans, miso, nuts, seeds, mushrooms, and broccoli. Unfortunately, grains, nuts, and seeds also contain phytic acid, which binds to zinc and prevents it from being absorbed.

- Pumpkin seeds are an excellent source of zinc and have a higher ratio of zinc to copper than other nuts and seeds. You can reduce their phytic acid content by soaking and roasting them.

Vitamin B$_6$ Supplementation

Supplementing with 200 to 800 mg of vitamin B$_6$ daily (in conjunction with zinc) has been found to result in dramatic reduction of pyroluria symptoms for most people (McGinnis et al. 2008b). I suggest starting with 100 mg of vitamin B$_6$ daily, increasing by 100 mg every two weeks, and monitoring your dream recall or nightmares throughout. You should notice your dreams becoming more frequent and pleasant each week. If urine testing confirms pyroluria, it's safe to supplement with up to 500 mg daily. I typically have my clients use 100 to 400 mg daily, and occasionally as much as 500 mg.

As with zinc, the RDA for vitamin B$_6$ is low: 2 mg or less. However, a good vitamin B complex will have at least 50 mg. Be aware that amounts of 50 mg or greater are considered to be a high amount, and you should reduce your dose if you notice any tingling in your fingers and other extremities. Called peripheral neuropathy, this can be a sign of too much vitamin B$_6$. But because vitamin B$_6$ is water soluble, this condition is completely reversible if you stop supplementing with vitamin B$_6$ or reduce your dose. If you find you need to lower your dose of vitamin B$_6$ but still aren't remembering your dreams, try taking pyridoxal 5-phosphate (P5P), starting with 25 mg daily. P5P is the active form of vitamin B$_6$ and is more absorbable. In fact, it's the only form some people can absorb. Because P5P is about four or five times more absorbable than vitamin B$_6$, 25 mg of P5P is equivalent to about 100 to 125 mg of vitamin B$_6$. Because P5P is more expensive and many of my clients do well on vitamin B$_6$, I always suggest starting with vitamin B$_6$.

As with all B vitamins, take vitamin B$_6$ and P5P with meals. They can be beneficial to take with lunch and dinner, because they play a role in production of serotonin, the "feel-good" neurotransmitter, and levels of serotonin tend to decline later in the day. However, you may find that taking them later in the day disrupts your sleep. If so, try taking them earlier. Here are some specific dosages and combinations you might try. Start with one, and if it works well for you, great! If not, continue to experiment with different combinations along these lines (to be clear, only use one of these regimens at a time):

- 100 to 500 mg of vitamin B_6

- 100 to 300 mg of vitamin B_6 and 25 to 50 mg of P5P

- 25 to 100 mg of P5P

You'll probably have to continue supplementing in this way indefinitely, although with time you may be able to reduce your dose. As mentioned, dream recall is a good indicator of your vitamin B_6 status, so you can use this as a way to determine whether you need to take more or less. Also keep in mind that you may need to increase your dose in times of stress. Vitamin B_6 can also be depleted by oral contraceptives, antidepressants, diuretics, or cortisone, so if you start or stop taking any of these, you may need to adjust the amount you supplement.

Aside from considerations about pyroluria, vitamin B_6 has been shown to be beneficial for helping with anxiety. This vitamin is important in the production of serotonin and GABA and therefore has a bearing on anxiety, depression, and pain (McCarty 2000). Vitamin B_6, together with magnesium, has proven helpful for anxiety associated with PMS (De Souza et al. 2000).

Food Sources of Vitamin B_6

As with zinc, it's good to try to get more vitamin B_6 from your diet, but if you do have pyroluria, you'll also need to supplement with vitamin B_6. Here are some of the best food sources:

- Grass-fed organic meat, pastured chickens and their eggs, and wild fish

- Vegetables, especially carrots, spinach, broccoli, and cabbage

- Whole grains, such as brown rice and quinoa

- Brewers yeast (high in all the B vitamins) and blackstrap molasses (also a good source of iron)

- Walnuts and sunflower seeds

- Alfalfa sprouts

Fatty Acids for Pyroluria

As discussed, people with pyroluria typically need to supplement with omega-6s, not omega-3s, so base any decision about supplementing on fatty acid testing. Here are some specific recommendations:

- 240 mg of GLA from evening primrose oil or borage oil, especially if fatty acid testing indicates a need for GLA

- Red meat, eggs, butter, and liver if fatty acid testing indicates low levels of arachidonic acid

- 1,000 mg of fish oil if fatty acid testing indicates a need for the omega-3s, which you can also get by eating oily fish like salmon, as well as walnuts; leafy, green vegetables; and ground flaxseeds or flaxseed oil

Other Nutrients for Pyroluria

Often, supplementing with zinc, vitamin B_6, and GLA will resolve the symptoms of pyroluria. If not, you may need to take 20 mg of manganese daily, as this mineral is often depleted in pyroluria and can be further depleted by supplementing with higher doses of zinc (Mathews-Larson 2001). Also include a B complex, on its own or in a multivitamin, to prevent a B vitamin imbalance. If you don't achieve complete relief from your symptoms by supplementing with all of these, you may need to consider taking the following supplements, as well (also covered in chapter 8):

- 1,000 to 3,000 mg of vitamin C

- 400 IU (international units) of vitamin E, as people with pyroluria often need higher amounts of antioxidants (McGinnis et al. 2008a, 2008b)

- 25 mg of iron, if you're anemic or have low ferritin (ibid.)

- 1,000 mg of vitamin B_3 (niacinamide), which is needed for serotonin synthesis and also helps reduce anxiety (Mathews-Larson 2001)

- 1,000 mg of vitamin B_5 (pantothenic acid), which supports the adrenal glands (ibid.)

- 400 mg of magnesium, which can become depleted when supplementing with large amounts of vitamin B_6 (ibid.)

Stress and Pyroluria

Pyroluria symptoms are made worse by stress, so it's important that you actively practice stress management, and chapter 8 has some excellent suggestions.

How Quickly You Can Expect Improvements

For mild to moderate pyroluria, supplementing with zinc, vitamin B_6, GLA, and manganese can lead to improvements in anxiety within one to two days, and even more progress within one week. For severe anxiety or those with other major imbalances or digestive problems, it can take a few weeks to a few months. Most people with pyroluria will have to continue supplementing indefinitely. If you stop taking the supplements, anxiety, social phobia, depression, stress, poor dream recall, and other symptoms can resurface within two to four weeks. You may need to take higher amounts of zinc and B_6 during times of illness, injury, or high stress.

As a side benefit, both zinc and vitamin B_6 help raise levels of serotonin, which will improve mood and sleep, and reduce afternoon and evening cravings.

CHAPTER 8

Other Nutrients, Hormone Imbalances, Toxins, Medications, and Lifestyle Changes

To fully resolve anxiety issues, you may need to consider taking a few other supplements. It may also be worthwhile to look at a few areas that are beyond the scope of nutrition, such as hormone imbalances, toxins, the effects of medications, and, last but not least, making some lifestyle changes.

Basic Supplements

It's important for everyone, anxious or not, to take a good multivitamin and multimineral with sufficient B vitamins and extra vitamin C, and iron if you need it (see the following section on iron). Combined with good-quality, real, whole food, these basics should keep you healthy. Supplementing with these nutrients is important because of the chemicals and toxins you're probably exposed to, as well as the stresses of everyday life. Plus, many minerals and B vitamins play a role in enzymatic processes and making neurotransmitters. As with any supplements you take, make sure these are of high quality and free of fillers, artificial colors, gluten, and other common allergens, such as soy and dairy.

A Multivitamin and Multimineral with B Vitamins

A good multivitamin and multimineral should contain all of the basic vitamins and minerals listed in the following table, which also provides general guidelines on amounts you should be taking. Getting adequate vitamin E, potassium, and selenium is particularly important, as deficiencies of these nutrients have been associated with anxiety and nervousness (Werbach 1999). You can find all of the following nutrients in a single supplement, but you could also buy three separate products: a multivitamin, a multimineral, and a B complex supplement. If you take a separate B complex supplement, look for a product with at least 50 mg of vitamins B_1, B_2, B_3, and B_6.

Nutrient	Daily intake
Vitamin A (as mixed carotenoids)	7,000 IU
Vitamin C (as ascorbic acid)	600 mg
Vitamin D (as cholecalciferol)	500 IU
Vitamin E (with mixed tocopherols)	100 IU
Vitamin B_1 (thiamine)	75 mg
Vitamin B_2 (riboflavin)	75 mg
Vitamin B_3 (niacinamide)	75 mg
Vitamin B_5 (pantothenic acid)	250 mg
Vitamin B_6 (pyridoxine)	50 mg
Vitamin B_{12} (as methylcobalamin)	500 mcg
Folic acid	400 mcg
Biotin	500 mcg
Calcium (chelated)	100 mg
Iodine (as kelp)	200 mcg
Magnesium (chelated)	200 mg
Zinc (chelated or OptiZinc)	30 mg
Selenium	250 mcg
Manganese (chelated)	1 mg
Chromium	200 mcg
Molybdenum	100 mcg
Potassium	100 mg
Choline	100 mg
Inositol	100 mg
PABA	25 mg
Boron	2 mg
Vanadium	100 mcg
Copper	1 mg

Iron

Typically, only young children and women who are menstruating need iron. However, iron-deficiency anemia (low iron), which is associated with apathy and depression (Benton and Donohoe 1999), is common, particularly in vegetarians (Baines, Powers, and Brown 2007) and women. I've seen low iron status in many of the anxious women I've worked with, as well as in those with pyroluria (see chapter 7), food sensitivities (see chapter 4), and digestive issues (see chapter 5). Sufficient iron is also needed for making the neurotransmitters serotonin and dopamine. However, excess iron can build up in the organs and be damaging, so look for supplements that don't contain iron unless you know you need it. The amount of iron in a multivitamin or multimineral is typically 8 mg. If you're anemic or have low serum ferritin, it's safe to take up to 25 mg daily (Pizzorno and Murray 2000). Iron supplements can cause nausea and constipation; to avoid these problems, look for a chelated form, such as iron bis-glycinate, which doesn't have this effect and is better absorbed than inorganic forms, like ferrous sulfate.

In terms of dietary sources, iron from animal sources (eggs, fish, liver, meat, and poultry) is absorbed better than iron from plant sources (leafy green vegetables, whole grains, blackstrap molasses, kelp, and legumes). A few simple dietary practices can enhance iron absorption: eating iron-rich foods together with foods high in vitamin C (such as tomatoes), using cast-iron cookware, and avoiding sugar. Certain dietary factors can also impair iron absorption: eating large amounts of foods that contain oxalic acid (chard, chocolate, kale, rhubarb, sorrel, spinach, and most nuts and beans); consuming dairy products, soft-drinks, high-sugar foods, coffee, and tea; having low levels of hydrochloric acid in the stomach; or taking fiber, calcium, vitamin E, zinc, or antacids at the same time as iron supplements.

Vitamin C

Mild to moderate deficiency of vitamin C may be associated with increased nervousness and anxiety (Heseker et al. 1992), and supplementing with vitamin C may be beneficial in times of stress

(Brody et al. 2002). This vitamin is an antioxidant, so it helps prevent damage by free radicals. It also boosts immunity and protects against toxins. You can safely take 1,000 to 3,000 mg of vitamin C a day, and I recommend that you take at least 3,000 mg a day in divided doses. Although you'll get some from your multivitamin, you'll need to take more to achieve this level. Look for a product that contains vitamin C as ascorbic acid. Good food sources of vitamin C include oranges, bell peppers, potatoes, strawberries, broccoli, and kale and other leafy greens.

Individual Nutrients for Anxiety

Several individual nutrients can also be beneficial for reducing anxiety and improving mood, including individual B vitamins, magnesium, calcium, vitamin D, omega-3 and omega-6 fatty acids, theanine, and lactium.

Extra B Vitamins

If you take individual B vitamins, also take a good B complex supplement to help prevent imbalances among these vitamins, which work together. Specific B vitamins have been shown to be deficient in patients with agoraphobia (Abbey 1982).

In a study of people with panic disorder, OCD, and depression, the B vitamin inositol in amounts of up to 18 grams daily was as effective and had fewer side effects than an antianxiety medication (Palatnik et al. 2001). This reflects my clinical experience, where I've found inositol to be very helpful with clients with obsessive and ruminating thoughts.

Vitamin B_1 is important for blood sugar control, and as you know from chapter 2, this has a major impact on anxiety. Vitamin B_3 is involved in many enzymatic processes and plays a key role in serotonin synthesis. At doses of 1,000 to 3,000 mg a day, it may be helpful for anxiety (Prousky 2004; Möhler et al. 1979). Vitamin B_5 is very important for the adrenals and therefore helps with modulating stress.

Folic acid and vitamin B_{12} are important for depression, and given the links between anxiety and depression, they may also be helpful for anxiety. They also support heart health, which is important if you suffer from anxiety or panic attacks, which stress the heart.

Good food sources of the B vitamins include liver, meat, turkey, whole grains, potatoes, bananas, chiles, legumes, nutritional yeast, and molasses.

Magnesium and Calcium

Magnesium is a calming mineral that nourishes the nervous system and helps prevent anxiety, fear, nervousness, restlessness, and irritability (Gaby 2004). Magnesium is also very protective of the heart and arteries (Seelig 1994); again, this is important if you suffer from anxiety or panic attacks. Supplemental magnesium, together with vitamin B_6, was shown to alleviate anxiety-related premenstrual symptoms, as well as breast tenderness and menstrual weight gain and pain (De Souza et al. 2000). This study also showed that even a small amount can make a difference; it used only 200 mg of magnesium and 50 mg of vitamin B_6. A typical supplemental amount is 400 to 600 mg of magnesium per day, usually with 800 to 1,200 mg of calcium, as it's typically best to get about twice as much calcium as magnesium. However, taking magnesium alone can be helpful for anxiety, and you may actually need more than the typical dose, perhaps as much as 1,000 mg of magnesium per day. Experiment with different amounts and decide what's right for you based on how you feel, and cut back if you get loose stools.

Taking magnesium and calcium at bedtime can also help promote restful sleep. A very pleasant and easy way to increase your intake of magnesium is to add about a cup of Epsom salts to a warm bath—you'll absorb the magnesium through your skin. Add some lavender essential oil and have a wonderful calming soak before bed, and you'll sleep better too.

Dark-green, leafy vegetables, like spinach, kale, and chard, contain plenty of calming magnesium as well as good amounts of the B vitamins. Whole, unrefined grains like oats, buckwheat, millet, and quinoa also contain both magnesium and B vitamins.

Other food sources of magnesium include legumes, beef, chicken, fish (especially halibut, cod, and salmon), nuts, seeds, bananas, watermelon, figs, potatoes, and green beans. Homemade bone broths (a favorite of mine) are rich in magnesium, calcium, and other vital minerals, with the added bonus that the gelatin in the broth enhances mineral absorption. Herbs are another source of magnesium. Try chamomile, dandelion, peppermint, or sage herbal tea; make a salad using fresh parsley, nettles, and dandelion; and add fennel seed, fenugreek, paprika, parsley, and cayenne when cooking.

Many high-magnesium foods are also a good source of calcium, especially spinach, turnip greens, mustard greens, collard greens, green beans, and sea vegetables. Other sources of calcium include dairy products, sardines, sesame seeds, broccoli, and celery. The herbs basil, thyme, rosemary, oregano, dill, and peppermint are also good sources of calcium, as is cinnamon.

Vitamin D

Vitamin D is a fat-soluble vitamin that is found in eggs and fatty fish such as salmon and mackerel (and cod liver oil), but your body can also make its own vitamin D after exposure to ultraviolet rays from the sun, though this is somewhat dependent on the season and your geographic location. It may improve seasonal anxiety and depression that worsen during the winter months (Lansdowne and Provost 1998). One study showed that vitamin D deficiency was associated with both anxiety and depression in fibromyalgia patients (Armstrong et al. 2007). Vitamin D is also important for immunity, bone health, and heart health, and it helps protect against cancer.

Recent research on vitamin D indicates that many people are deficient in this key vitamin. I recommend that all of my clients have their vitamin D levels checked and have found that the majority have low levels. Vitamin D status can be measured by a simple blood test, 25-hydroxy-vitamin D. Dr. John Cannell, founder of the Vitamin D Council, considers the new vitamin D guidelines released in November 2010—600 IU for adults up to age seventy—to be too low (Cannell 2010). He recommends taking 5,000 IU daily until your level is between 50 and 80 ng/mL (nanograms per milliliter), the midpoint of the current lab reference range of 32 to 100 ng/mL.

Don't be surprised if your doctor prescribes 50,000 IU per week. Once your levels are ideal, a typical maintenance dose ranges from 2,000 to 5,000 IU per day. It's a good idea to test your level every three months. When supplementing, be sure to take vitamin D_3 (cholecalciferol). Vitamin D_2 (ergocalciferol) is the synthetic form and not effective. Recent research suggests that it's most effective to take vitamin D with your largest meal (Mulligan and Licata 2010). Also, keep in mind that a great deal of research is being conducted on the health benefits of vitamin D, and it's a controversial topic, so recommendations in regard to ideal level, dose, and timing may change. The Vitamin D Council is a good resource for recent findings.

Omega-3s and Omega-6s

It's well-known that omega-3s from fish oil (EPA and DHA) are effective for alleviating depression, and one study looking at substance abusers with low fish consumption found that supplementing with fish oil for three months resulted in less anxiety and anger (Buydens-Branchey, Branchey, and Hibbeln 2008). I recommend that you eat fish, including some oily fish, such as salmon and sardines, and only supplement with fish oil if you know for sure that your levels of omega-3s are low. A good starting dose is 1,000 mg daily. Fatty acids tests are available from labs such as Metametrix; results will indicate whether you need to supplement with omega-3s, omega-6s, or both, and will also indicate your levels of damaging trans fats. Many anxious people with pyroluria don't need to supplement with omega-3s but do seem to need the omega-6 GLA, ideally in the form of evening primrose oil (see chapter 7 for more on this topic).

Theanine and Lactium

L-theanine, an amino acid found in tea, has a calming effect and reduces physiological responses to stress (Kimura et al. 2007). It also raises levels of GABA, the calming neurotransmitter. It also has properties that offer protection against environmental neurotoxins (Cho et al. 2008). A typical supplemental dose of theanine is 50 to 200 mg.

Lactium, a supplement made from the casein protein in milk, has been shown to reduce stress-related symptoms, including anxiety, emotional and social problems, and digestive issues (Kim et al. 2007). This product also lowers levels of the stress hormone cortisol. It has been very effective for some of my anxious clients who don't benefit from supplementing with calming amino acids. A typical supplemental dose of lactium is 150 mg per day.

Hormone Imbalances

Hormone imbalances are beyond the scope of nutrition solutions, but you may need to consider them as part of a holistic plan for dealing with anxiety and stress. Hormones are complex, and you'll need to work with a holistic health practitioner to address adrenal dysfunction, thyroid problems, and sex hormone imbalances, so I'll just address these topics briefly to help you get a sense of whether any of these hormone imbalances could be affecting you. For further reading, a good resource is *The Phytogenic Hormone Solution* (2002), by Saundra McKenna.

Adrenal Dysfunction

The adrenal glands are responsible for helping the body deal with stress of any kind—physical, mental, or emotional. They initiate and moderate the fight-or-flight response, which can be triggered simply by perceiving something as a threat, even if it isn't actually threatening. In our modern, faced-paced era, the adrenals are often overworked, particularly among people with anxiety, which can heighten the perception of threat posed by everyday situations.

One of the key stress hormones produced by the adrenals is cortisol. A certain amount of cortisol is essential. When stress isn't an issue, cortisol is produced in a distinctive pattern, with levels highest in the morning, dropping slightly around lunchtime, dropping a little more around dinnertime, and then at their lowest at bedtime so you can get a good night's sleep.

Chronic stress leads to chronic overproduction of cortisol, which can cause a variety of problems. You may have elevated levels of cortisol at various times or a disrupted cortisol production pattern. If this goes on too long, the adrenals can become fatigued and produce too little cortisol. Any of these may worsen anxiety or depression. The adrenals have other important functions. For example, they produce sex hormones, and for women, they become a key source of sex hormones when ovarian production of these hormones diminishes at menopause, so it's important that the adrenals be in good shape.

There are many signs and symptoms of adrenal fatigue, including allergies (food or environmental), carbohydrate sensitivity, low immunity, poor blood sugar control, and feeling constantly drained and exhausted. Symptoms of elevated cortisol include sleep problems and a "wired-tired" feeling.

Saliva tests that measure your cortisol levels at different points in the day are the best assessment tool, as they will indicate your daily production pattern. The Adrenal Stress Index test by Diagnos-Techs is an example.

For adrenal fatigue, addressing stress is crucial. Be sure to read the recommendations on relaxation, vacations, and sleep later in this chapter, and to try a variety of de-stressing techniques to find what works best for you. It's important to also address physical sources of stress, such as food sensitivities, dysbiosis, and toxins. Specific nutrients and herbs can help heal the adrenals: vitamin C, B complex, extra vitamin B_5, licorice, ashwagandha, and holy basil. Adrenal glandular products (like Isocort) can provide your body with cortisol while your adrenals are recovering and healing. If cortisol levels are elevated, phosphorylated serine and lactium can help lower them.

Thyroid Dysfunction

A well-functioning thyroid gland is important for the metabolic activity of every cell in the body. And because thyroid hormones play such a key role in the functioning of the entire endocrine system, an underactive thyroid, or hypothyroidism, can go hand in hand with adrenal fatigue and sex hormone imbalances.

Common symptoms of low thyroid function include low energy, sensitivity to cold, depression, PMS, memory problems, dry skin, weight gain, and constipation. Often there is a family history of thyroid problems. Hypothyroidism can diminish the effectiveness of supplemental amino acids for balancing brain chemistry, so if you tried the approaches in chapter 6 and didn't benefit appreciably, it would be good to have your levels of thyroid hormones checked. Blood tests for thyroid health should include TSH (thyroid-stimulating hormone), free T3 (triiodothyronine), free T4 (thyroxine), reverse T3, and thyroid antibodies (antithyroglobulin and antithyroperoxidase). Elevated levels of thyroid antibodies may indicate an autoimmune condition called Hashimoto's thyroiditis, which can result in fluctuations of thyroid hormones that may sometimes cause a racing heart and other symptoms that feel like anxiety (similar to symptoms of an overactive thyroid, or hyperthyroidism). If you do have elevated thyroid antibodies, you need to avoid grains that contain gluten (Duntas 2009). (See chapter 4 for more on the connection between celiac disease and Hashimoto's thyroiditis.)

Soy products suppress thyroid function, as do raw cruciferous vegetables, such as cauliflower, cabbage, Brussels sprouts, broccoli, and many dark, leafy greens. I suggest avoiding soy and eating the majority of your cruciferous vegetables cooked, as this destroys the compounds that adversely affect the thyroid. Toxins that can impair thyroid function include fluoride, bromide, and chlorine. Some medications can also impair thyroid function, including estrogen, birth control pills, and lithium.

Nutrients that help support the thyroid include tyrosine, selenium, iodine (found in fish and sea vegetables), vitamin A, ashwagandha, and zinc.

Because of the way adrenal function and thyroid function are interrelated, it's best to address any adrenal problems using the suggestions above and work with a holistic practitioner to find the right combination of thyroid support: nutrients, desiccated thyroid products such as Armour or Nature-Throid, medications, or a combination.

Sex Hormone Imbalances in Women

If your adrenal or thyroid function is impaired, you may also need to have your levels of sex hormones tested. All of the elements of the endocrine system—hormones and the glands that secrete them—are interrelated in a complex system of checks and balances. I like to say they all do this merry little dance together. Having one element of the system out of balance can create a cascade of effects that impair other components of the system.

As for specific effects and symptoms of sex hormone imbalances, low progesterone levels are often associated with high levels of copper and low zinc, and therefore increased anxiety, depression, and mood swings. Other signs of low progesterone include irregular menstrual cycles and PMS, insomnia, headaches, irritability, weight gain and cravings, fluid retention, and frequent urination. Low levels of estrogen lead to low levels of serotonin, which can lead to anxiety and depression. Other signs of low estrogen include hot flashes, night sweats, fatigue, low libido, vaginal dryness, and poor mental function.

Diagnos-Techs offers several salivary tests that can assess levels of sex hormones. The specifics of the tests vary, including when samples are collected, which for women depends on whether you're menstruating regularly, in perimenopause, or menopausal.

Reduce Your Exposure to Toxins

Most of us are exposed to a wide array of toxins on a daily basis. Heavy metals are of particular concern because of their neurological effects. Unfortunately some exposure to toxins is simply unavoidable. However, you can do quite a bit to reduce your exposure by drinking filtered water and making some straightforward changes at home, as well as supporting your liver, the primary detoxification organ (see chapter 5).

Toxins in the Home

If you're like most people, you're surrounded by toxins even at home. They're in plastics, nonstick cookware, paint, carpeting, furniture, household cleaning products, and even personal care products such as shampoo and lotions. If you're on a municipal water system, your tap water also contains toxins, including chlorine and fluoride. Because toxins can affect your nervous system, your organs, and your hormones, they may contribute to anxiety.

There are some great books on avoiding toxins in your home. For starters, I recommend *Home Safe Home* (1997), by Debra Lynn Dadd. She has wonderful nontoxic suggestions for everything from sheets and floor coverings to cleaning products and office supplies. Another great resource is the Environmental Working Group. They have an excellent website with information about the effects of toxins on health and much more. They also have a database where you can look up safety ratings of personal care products and their ingredients. Though the brand of shampoo you use may seem innocuous, it might have a high toxicity rating due to the fragrance (neurotoxic and allergenic) or methylparaben (allergenic, toxic to the organs, a skin irritant, and an endocrine disruptor). Clearing out the toxins will be good for you emotionally and physically—and it will also be good for the earth!

Heavy Metals

Heavy metals should always be considered with mood problems, especially if the other solutions in this book haven't helped you with your anxiety. We all have some level of exposure to heavy metals, and some of us are more susceptible to their effects than others. Mercury from environmental sources, high-mercury fish, or amalgam dental fillings can have an effect on mental health, leading to feelings of anxiety and agitation, as well as problems with concentration and many physical symptoms (O'Carroll et al. 1995; Kidd 2000). Lead may also be an issue, and even low levels in the blood may be implicated in anxiety, panic attacks, and depression (Bouchard et al. 2009).

Urine tests for heavy metals (offered by Metametrix) can identify your levels of heavy metals, and the porphyrins test will also give an indication of resulting ill effects. Hair analysis by Analytical Research Labs shows levels of heavy metals (and whether you're excreting them), as well as levels of several minerals.

Various detoxification programs can help you reduce your heavy metal load. If you suspect heavy metal exposure, I recommend doing a gentle, nutrient-dense functional liver detoxification program, described in chapter 5, a few times a year, and working with a health professional who specializes in this area.

Understand the Effects of Medications

Medications have side effects and can also cause nutrient depletions, both of which can make anxiety worse. Try to find the root cause of health problems and use natural solutions if possible. If you currently take medications, work with your doctor to find ways to reduce your dose or stop taking them altogether. This may mean finding a doctor who's more open to alternative approaches. Keep in mind Pfeiffer's law, proposed by physician and biochemist Carl Pfeiffer, which states that "for every drug that benefits a patient, there is a natural substance that can achieve the same effect" (Walsh 1991, 4).

Certain medications (both prescription and nonprescription) may cause restlessness, nervousness, insomnia, and other symptoms of anxiety. They include decongestants, steroids such as cortisone and prednisone, respiratory medications such as albuterol, weight-loss products, high blood pressure medications, attention deficit/hyperactivity disorder medications, birth control pills, antidepressants, and thyroid medications. If you do take medications, always read the side effects insert so that you'll know what to watch for. A good Internet source for information on medications and side effects is MedlinePlus.

Here are a few examples of side effects related to anxiety: Prozac and Prempro list nervousness as a side effect, Sudafed lists restlessness, Ritalin lists nervousness and restlessness, and Synthroid lists tremors, insomnia, and nervousness. A more serious side effect of many antidepressants is increased risk of suicide. Another consideration is the additives and fillers in medications, such as wheat, corn, and artificial colors. If you're sensitive to them, they may cause problems even in small amounts.

It's also important to be aware that many medications can deplete your body of specific nutrients. Here are a few examples (Pelton, LaValle, and Hawkins 2001): Vitamin B_6 is depleted by oral contraceptives, decongestants, and antidepressants. Other B vitamins are also depleted by oral contraceptives. Zinc is depleted by corticosteroids, ACE inhibitors, and oral contraceptives. Magnesium is depleted by many medications. As you may have noticed, all of these nutrients are important for preventing and eliminating anxiety.

The class of drugs called benzodiazepines, frequently prescribed for anxiety, should be used only short term, yet many people continue taking them for years. Some examples are Ativan, Klonopin, and Valium. Because of their addictive nature and because tolerance for these tranquilizers increases over time, withdrawing from them can cause extremely unpleasant psychological and physical symptoms, including anxiety and panic attacks, muscle pain, and headaches. A good resource for learning more about these medications and how to taper off your dosage is www.benzo.org.uk, a website dedicated to helping people avoid or recover from benzodiazepine addiction. Anxiety is an extremely common adverse effect of withdrawal from virtually all psychiatric medications, including SSRIs. It may be dangerous and uncomfortable to stop these medications abruptly, and this should be done under the care of a nutritionally oriented physician who can taper your medication slowly while being open to your receiving nutritional support.

Statin drugs are of particular concern. With all of the bad press cholesterol receives, you may find the next point surprising, but it's true: if your cholesterol levels are too low, you're at increased risk for anxiety, depression, and even suicide. One study (Suarez 1999) found a relationship between low cholesterol and increased anxiety and depression in women. And when total cholesterol is less than 160 mg/dl (milligrams per deciliter), there may be an increased risk of suicide (Perez-Rodriguez et al. 2008). An interesting article in the journal *Circulation* reported that these same levels were also associated with increased risk of death from strokes, cancer, and digestive and respiratory diseases (Hulley, Walsh, and Newman 1992). In addition, that article emphasized that, among women, there is no association between high blood cholesterol and cardiovascular deaths. This suggests that statins, used to lower cholesterol, shouldn't be so widely prescribed for women.

Make Important Lifestyle Changes

Although the lifestyle changes discussed in this chapter are outside of the realm of food, they're important in a holistic approach to anxiety. You need to support the hard and important work of making dietary changes, balancing blood sugar and brain chemistry, and addressing nutrient deficiencies with a few key changes in other areas of life: getting enough exercise, getting enough sleep, considering therapy or a support group, and setting aside time for relaxation.

Do Some Exercise, Preferably Outdoors

Exercise has seemingly endless benefits for both physical and mental health, with many studies supporting that it can help with anxiety, stress, depression, and addictive behaviors (Petruzzello et al. 1991; Tkachuk and Martin 1999). An interesting study from the Netherlands found a strong relationship between being outdoors in nature and lower rates of anxiety and depression (and other diseases), especially in children and in poorer communities (Jolanda et al. 2009). Plus, both exercise and sunshine raise serotonin levels, which may be low when you have anxiety. So I recommend that you put these two together and increase the benefits of physical activity by exercising outdoors. This could be anything from a gentle walk in the fresh air and sunshine to tennis, mountain biking, or windsurfing. The key is to find something you enjoy; otherwise you won't stick with it.

Get Enough Sleep

There's evidence supporting a correlation between mood disorders, including anxiety and depression, and sleep disturbances (van Mill et al. 2010). Beyond that, poor sleep has a large impact on overall health. It's important to get enough sleep; for most people, that means eight to nine hours a night. However, a recent poll (National Sleep Foundation 2009) found that only 28 percent of those surveyed regularly got eight hours or more of sleep a night.

The average was around six and a half hours on weekdays and seven on weekends. Those who slept less than eight hours a night typically had mood problems, including worry and anxiety, ate more sugar and unhealthy food, drank more caffeinated beverages, used more tobacco, and exercised less.

If you have both anxiety and sleep problems, resolving your anxiety could take care of your insomnia, because they may both have the same underlying cause. For example, they could be related to low levels of serotonin and melatonin or low levels of GABA (see chapter 6). Or they could be related to high levels of cortisol or low blood sugar at night, in which case supporting the adrenals will help (see chapter 2 and earlier sections of this chapter). It's also important to look at food sensitivities (see chapter 4), avoiding caffeine and alcohol (see chapter 3), digestion (see chapter 5), and mineral deficiencies (see earlier sections of this chapter), as these can also affect sleep.

Here are some sleep tips that may also help, in addition to addressing the previous issues:

- Sleep in a completely dark room. If this isn't possible, try wearing a travel eye mask.

- If noise is a problem, wear earplugs. This can be especially helpful when you're traveling and surrounded by strange sounds.

- Don't watch TV or use the computer just before bed.

- During the day, exercise to raise serotonin levels, and get some bright sunlight to boost your melatonin production at night.

- Take a warm, relaxing bath before bed, with Epsom salts and a few drops of lavender oil.

- Near bedtime, try drinking some relaxing chamomile tea.

- Be in bed by 10 p.m.

- Keep your bedroom cool.

- Reserve your bed for two things: sleeping and making love.

- Try some of the relaxation techniques discussed later in the chapter.

Consider Therapy and Support Groups

There are entire books on the benefits of therapy and support groups, so I won't go into details here. But I do want to stress that these approaches are extremely helpful. One very effective method for anxiety is cognitive behavior therapy, which aims to help people overcome unworkable thinking patterns and habitual behaviors. Eye movement desensitization and reprocessing (EMDR) may also be helpful. There are many excellent anxiety workbooks available by psychologist and anxiety expert Edmund Bourne. He has also coauthored a super book titled *Natural Relief for Anxiety* (Bourne, Brownstein, and Garano 2004).

Set Aside Time for Relaxation

For many of my clients, simply relaxing is one of the hardest things to do. Yet it's so important to slow down, say no, get help, and set aside time for relaxation in a variety of forms, from vacations to proven relaxation techniques like yoga, tai chi, and meditation. You can't just say you'll slow down or say you'll relax by watching TV. You also need to do something planned that really fosters relaxation and rejuvenation. Being on overdrive day after day, with too many things on your plate, too many commitments, and expectations that are too high, is a setup for fatigue, stress, anxiety, worry, burnout, and possibly failure. Don't feel overwhelmed by all of the options below; you need not try them all. Just pick a few and do what works for you.

Take Up Yoga, Tai Chi, Qigong, or Meditation

Yoga, tai chi, qigong, and meditation all provide many physical and emotional benefits. In one study, yoga, breath work, and meditation enhanced mood, reduced stress and anxiety, and enhanced mental focus (Brown and Gerbarg 2005). Yoga has been shown to raise GABA levels (Streeter et al. 2007), and meditation raises serotonin levels (Bujatti and Riederer 1976). Levels of both of these neurotransmitters can be low when you're anxious. (See chapter 6 for more on GABA and serotonin.) Kundalini yoga meditation techniques have been found to be effective for obsessive-compulsive disorder (OCD) and may also be helpful with fear, phobias, and other anxiety disorders, as well as depression, addictions, and insomnia (Shannahoff-Khalsa 2004). In a review of studies of the effects of tai chi and qigong among older adults (Rogers, Larkey, and Keller 2009), these practices were found to help with anxiety and depression, improve physical function, and reduce blood pressure and the risk of falling.

Take a Real Vacation Every Year

Americans take the shortest vacations in the industrial world: thirteen days a year, compared to twenty-one or more in Canada, Britain, Germany, and South Africa. There aren't many studies on the benefits of vacations and none that look specifically at anxiety. But vacations do seem to have positive effects on health and well-being (de Bloom et al. 2009), even if these benefits only last a short while. They can also improve mood and sleep and lessen physical complaints (Strauss-Blasche, Ekmekcioglu, and Marktl 2000). By definition, a vacation is leisure time that doesn't involve work and that's devoted to rest or pleasure. So do something where you get to have fun, relax, sleep, and eat great, nourishing food. And, for additional mood benefits, get out in nature and sunshine and be active. Taking a week off to paint your house doesn't count as a vacation!

Try Guided Imagery

Guided imagery involves using positive thoughts and images to help bring about change and healing. Many studies support its benefits for anxiety, panic attacks, stress, and depression (Apóstolo and Kolcaba 2009). It can also help with many other conditions, including insomnia and pain (Stiefel and Stagno 2004), and addictions (Avants and Margolin 1995). My favorite resource for this is recordings by Belleruth Naparstek, available from Health Journeys (see resources). She has a gentle, calming voice and uses wonderful imagery to help you feel calm and relaxed.

Other Techniques That May Help

There are some simple practices and techniques that can be very calming and relaxing:

- Massage has many health benefits and can also help with stress and anxiety (Rho et al. 2006).

- Essential oils such as lavender, rose, orange, bergamot, lemon, sandalwood, clary sage, and chamomile can be very calming (Setzer 2009). They can be used in aromatherapy, added to a bath or massage oils, or dabbed on the wrists.

- Based on the limited research, acupuncture appears to be beneficial for some forms of anxiety (Pilkington et al. 2007).

- Try relaxation exercises such as progressive and passive muscle relaxation, and get into the habit of doing abdominal breathing. These techniques are described in *Natural Relief for Anxiety* (Bourne, Brownstein, and Garano 2004).

- You might also try the emotional freedom technique, which involves tapping on acupuncture points while focusing on the issue at hand (Benor et al. 2009).

- And always remember that laughter is wonderful for relieving stress and anxiety and improving your overall mood. Watch a funny movie, find something joyful to do, and have fun!

Parting Words

I hope this book has inspired you, encouraged you, and given you plenty of information and tools to help you use the amazing healing powers of food and nutrients, along with lifestyle changes, to calm your anxious mind, and also improve your mood and end cravings. This book is just the start. I encourage you to become an expert in your own situation by experimenting and observing, and to continue to learn more about nutrition and health as well. Attend workshops offered by nutritionists, chiropractors, naturopathic doctors, and other holistic health practitioners. Watch educational movies and read books that teach about foods and their health benefits. Enjoy, explore, and become inspired. New information is always becoming available, so remember to check this book's website (www.anti anxietyfoodsolution.com) from time to time for more resources to help you along the way.

Know that you are not alone. Connect with friends, family, or a support group and share how you feel. Also share what you've learned. This is a great way to take ownership of what you've learned while also helping others. And always remember that there's no shame in having a mental disorder. You really can feel on top of the world!

APPENDIX 1

Sue's Story

All of the case studies throughout the book are real examples of people I've worked with. Their stories demonstrate that we are all different, so we each need to figure out what our own unique nutritional needs are to determine what changes are needed. You may just need to make changes to your diet, or you may need to do more. I include the following case study here, because for this client the solution involved multiple approaches, covered throughout the book. Her story also shows the diversity of reasons for anxiety, and therefore the need for flexibility in approaches to alleviating it, and highlights the importance of finding the root cause of the issue, whether it's eating poorly, not eating frequently enough, caffeine, poor digestion, gluten issues, or pyroluria.

Sue's situation was more complex than that of most of my clients. She needed more testing and, ultimately, more supplements. A stay-at-home mom in her forties who played the violin in a community orchestra, Sue was anxious and experienced weekly panic attacks related to her musical performances. She typically felt anxious throughout the day, especially around bedtime. She said that she'd always been anxious but that her anxiety had gotten worse in the last year. She was also tired and mildly depressed, and had pretty severe PMS, including bloating and emotional symptoms, especially tearfulness. She had major cravings for bread, pasta, and fats, with her absolute-favorite foods being big chunks of French bread with plenty of butter and pasta with creamy sauces. She said she *loved* these foods. Other than this, she ate fairly well, mostly eating a whole foods diet, with sufficient high-quality protein, good fats, and organic vegetables and fruit.

During our first appointment, I recommended that Sue take 250 mg of GABA for its relaxing effects. She immediately felt a sense of calm. She was visibly more relaxed and much more at ease. Because Sue had a number of symptoms of low serotonin (mild depression, winter blues and anxiety, perfectionism, afternoon cravings, and PMS), I also recommended that she try 50 mg of 5-HTP. The results were dramatic. Within ten minutes she felt more positive.

Because of her intense love for bread and pasta, I suspected that Sue also had low levels of endorphins. I recommended that she take D-phenylalanine (DPA) and a supplemental free-form amino acid blend to help raise her endorphins so that she wouldn't need to turn to food to self-soothe.

Sue had a very high score on the pyroluria questionnaire. She didn't recall her dreams, indicating a need for vitamin B_6. And when I had her do the zinc taste test, she didn't think the zinc solution had any taste, indicating a high need for zinc. I recommended that she take the following supplements, and she agreed to give it a try:

- A multivitamin with chromium

- A multimineral

- A B complex supplement

- 1,000 mg of vitamin C three times a day

- 50 mg of 5-HTP at midmorning and 100 mg of 5-HTP at midafternoon

- 250 mg of GABA on waking and at midmorning, and 250 to 500 mg at midafternoon and bedtime

- 1,000 mg of DPA at midmorning and midafternoon

- A free-form amino acid blend with every meal

- 30 mg of zinc

- 100 mg of vitamin B_6

At my recommendation, she had the tests for a wide variety of potential problems: IgG food allergies (including gluten), adrenal dysfunction, pyroluria, fatty acid deficiencies, and sex hormone imbalances. I also recommended basic blood work to determine her levels of vitamin D, ferritin, cholesterol, and so on. Given her mood problems and her craving for bread and pasta, I also recommended that she do a two-week gluten elimination-challenge trial, and she said she'd start right away.

The week after her first appointment, Sue had no panic attacks— not a single one. She was thrilled and told me, "For the first time in a long while, I have hope." She was feeling much less overwhelmed and more optimistic, and was sleeping well. However, she was still tired, and although her cravings were less intense, they were still a problem. I suggested she double her 5-HTP to help with the cravings, and this worked.

A week later, when Sue added gluten back into her diet, she felt more tired, spacey, and moody, and also slightly more anxious. Then her lab tests came in, confirming her sensitivity to gluten, along with a large number of other foods. Given the results she'd already seen from cutting out gluten, Sue readily agreed to remove all of the problem foods from her diet.

The adrenal testing confirmed low cortisol levels and adrenal fatigue, so Sue started taking a general adrenal support supplement and extra vitamin B_5. The fatty acid testing indicated low levels across the board, possibly due to poor absorption as a result of gut damage due to food sensitivities. I recommended that Sue start taking supplemental omega-3s in the form of fish oil and omega-6s as evening primrose oil, and encouraged her to use more olive oil and coconut oil in her cooking.

Sue's tests also confirmed that she had pyroluria, confirming the need for zinc and vitamin B_6. On top of all of this, her lab tests also showed that she was anemic, a problem that commonly co-occurs with gluten sensitivity and pyroluria, so Sue started taking supplemental iron. Her progesterone level was also low, but we decided to wait a few cycles to see if this would improve as a result of all the other interventions.

Six weeks after her first appointment, Sue's energy had improved, and she was excited to experiment with more adventurous endeavors in the kitchen, such as using more fermented foods and making her own sprouts. By now the liquid zinc was tasting strong, and she was remembering her dreams. During a particularly stressful time, she stopped remembering her dreams, so she increased her vitamin B_6 for a short while and soon started remembering them again. She also realized that she was much more relaxed and less perfectionistic. Given all of her improvements, I recommended that she quit taking GABA except during stressful times, and this worked well for her.

Eventually, Sue was able to start tapering off the supplemental amino acids, but she kept taking the basic supplements, zinc, and vitamin B_6. She decided to continue avoiding gluten but was able to reintroduce many of the other problem foods on a rotational basis. At three months after her first appointment, Sue's mood was great, her cravings were entirely gone, and she'd lost fifteen pounds. She had good energy, was sleeping well, and didn't have any PMS in her last menstrual cycle. And, remarkably, she hadn't had a single panic attack since her first appointment.

APPENDIX 2

Food, Mood, Energy, Cravings, and Sleep Log

This log will help you get a better understanding of how your mood, energy, cravings, and sleep are affected by your diet and any supplements you take. It's helpful to keep a food log anytime, but especially whenever you're experimenting with avoiding certain foods, adding foods to your diet, taking new supplements, and making other dietary changes. When using the food log, record everything you eat and when. Also keep track of the supplements you take. The fifth column is the key. Use it to describe how you feel after eating or taking supplements, in terms of mood (anxious or calm, sad or happy, and so on), your energy level, whether you experience cravings and how severe they are, and the quality of your sleep. You may find it helpful to rate all of these aspects over the course of the day. You could use a scale of 1 to 10, with 10 being optimum; for example, great mood = 9, or medium energy = 5. For menstruating women, fluctuating hormone levels could have an effect, so also record the day of your cycle, with the first day of your period being day 1. Also keep track of your digestion and bowel movements (BMs).

Food, Mood, Energy, Cravings and Sleep Log

Date:

Cycle Day:

Time	Food or beverages	Supplements	Mood, energy, cravings, and sleep (score out of 10)	Digestion / BMs
	Breakfast:			
	Snack:			
	Lunch:			
	Snack:			
	Dinner:			
	Snack:			

Resources

Internet Resources

The Antianxiety Food Solution (www.antianxietyfoodsolution .com). The website for this book, with new research results, additional case studies, summary checklists for each chapter, an index, additional resources, and new information as it becomes available.

Benzodiazapine Addiction, Withdrawal, and Recovery (benzo.org.uk). An organization dedicated to helping people avoid or recover from addiction to benzodiazepines, a class of drugs frequently prescribed for anxiety.

Citizens for Health (www.citizens.org). The voice of the natural health consumer and pioneers in the natural health freedom movement, providing valuable information about healthy food, complementary approaches to health, and nontoxic products.

Environmental Working Group (ewg.org). Great information about pesticides and toxins in water and cleaning products, and much more, including a database with information on the safety of various body-care products (cosmeticdatabase.com).

Every Woman Over 29 (everywomanover29.com). The website of my nutrition practice, with newsletter, programs, workshops, blog, and additional resources.

Health Journeys (healthjourneys.com). Guided imagery recordings by Belleruth Naparstek, with many titles to help with stress and promote well-being.

Holistic Moms Network (www.holisticmoms.org). A national nonprofit connecting parents who are interested in holistic health and green living, with a super forum and wonderful local meetings.

Institute for Responsible Technology (responsibletechnology .org). Information about genetically modified food and its health and environmental consequences.

LocalHarvest (www.localharvest.org). Directory of local farms, farmers' markets, and CSAs (community supported agriculture).

MedlinePlus (www.nlm.nih.gov/medlineplus/druginformation.html). A service of the U.S. National Library of Medicine and National Institutes of Health that offers information on medications and their side effects.

Monterey Bay Aquarium (montereybayaquarium.org). Offers good information about healthful and environmentally sound choices in seafood at their website's Seafood Watch section, along with pocket guides for when you go shopping.

National Association of Nutrition Professionals (nanp.org). Find a nutrition professional to guide you, find a nutrition school to attend, find a chef, and more.

The Specific Carbohydrate Diet (breakingtheviciouscycle.info). Information on the Specific Carbohydrate Diet (SCD).

U.S. Wellness Meats (www.grasslandbeef.com). A mail-order source for grass-fed meat and other wonderful products like pemmican, if you can't get them locally. They support family farms, sustainable farming, and humane practices.

Vital Choice (www.vitalchoice.com). Mail-order source for wild, sustainable, and delicious salmon and other seafood, if you can't get them locally.

Weston A. Price Foundation (westonaprice.org). Education about nutrient-dense traditional foods and more, with a great annual conference.

Lab Tests

Analytical Research Labs
arltma.com
2225 W. Alice Ave.
Phoenix, AZ 85021
800-528-4067

Offers hair analysis testing for heavy metals and mineral levels.

Diagnos-Techs Clinical and Research Laboratory
diagnostechs.com
19110 66th Ave. S., Bldg. G
Kent, WA 98032
800-878-3787

Offers a number of tests, including salivary sex hormone tests, stool tests, and the Adrenal Stress Index (ASI) salivary test, which measures cortisol four times during the day, as well as DHEA, secretory immunoglobulin A, and antigliadin antibodies.

EnteroLab
www.enterolab.com
10875 Plano Rd., Ste. 123
Dallas, TX 75238
972-686-6869

Offers stool testing for gluten sensitivity and HLA-DQ2 and HLA-DQ8 gene testing.

Health Diagnostics and Research Institute (formerly Vitamin Diagnostics)

> europeanlaboratory.com
> 540 Bordentown Ave., Suite 2300
> South Amboy, NJ 08879
> 732-721-1234

Offers many tests, including urine pyroluria/kryptopyrrole (in 2011), whole blood histamine, fatty acids, and platelet neurotransmitters (serotonin and catecholamines).

Metametrix Clinical Lab

> metametrix.com
> 3425 Corporate Way
> Duluth, GA 30096
> 800-221-4640

Offers many tests, including the GI Effects stool test, Comprehensive Metabolic Profile, organic acids testing, celiac panels, and IgG food antibodies in both a serum test (blood draw) and a finger-prick version, as well as urine and porphyrin testing for heavy metals.

Recommended Reading

Nutritional Healing

Blaylock, R. L. 1997. *Excitotoxins: The Taste That Kills.* Santa Fe, NM: Health Press.

Bourne, E. J., A. Brownstein, and L. Garano. 2004. *Natural Relief for Anxiety: Complementary Strategies for Easing Fear, Panic, and Worry.* Oakland, CA: New Harbinger Publications.

Braly, J., and R. Hoggan. 2002. *Dangerous Grains: Why Gluten Cereal Grains May Be Hazardous to Your Health.* New York: Penguin Putnam.

Braverman, E. R. 2003. *The Healing Nutrients Within.* Laguna Beach, CA: Basic Health Publications.

Campbell-McBride, N. 2008. *Gut and Psychology Syndrome: Natural Treatment for Autism, ADD/ADHD, Dyslexia, Dyspraxia,*

Depression, Schizophrenia. Cambridge, UK: Medinform Publishing.

Cass, H., and P. Holford. 2002. *Natural Highs: Feel Good All the Time.* New York: Penguin.

Cordain, L. 2001. *The Paleo Diet: Lose Weight and Get Healthy by Eating the Food You Were Designed to Eat.* Hoboken, NJ: Wiley.

Edelman, E. 2001. *Natural Healing for Schizophrenia and Other Common Mental Disorders.* Eugene, OR: Borage Books.

Hoffer, A., and M. Walker. 1996. *Putting It All Together: The New Orthomolecular Nutrition.* New Canaan, CT: Keats Publishing.

Hyman, M. 2009. *The UltraMind Solution: Fixing Your Broken Brain by Healing Your Body First.* New York: Simon and Schuster.

Jacobs, G. 1997. *Beat Candida Through Diet.* London: Random House.

Lipski, E. 2004. *Digestive Wellness.* New York: McGraw Hill.

Mathews-Larson, J. 2001. *Depression-Free Naturally: 7 Weeks to Eliminating Anxiety, Despair, Fatigue, and Anger from Your Life.* New York: Random House.

McKenna, S. 2002. *The Phytogenic Hormone Solution.* New York: Random House.

Pfeiffer, C. 1987. *Nutrition and Mental Illness.* Rochester, VT: Healing Arts Press.

Prousky, J. E. 2006. *Anxiety: Orthomolecular Diagnosis and Treatment.* Ottawa, Ontario, Canada: CCNM Press.

Ross, J. 2004. *The Mood Cure: The 4-Step Program to Take Charge of Your Emotions—Today.* New York: Penguin.

Ross, J. 2011. The *Diet Cure: The 8-Step Program to Rebalance Your Body Chemistry, End Food Cravings, Weight Problems, and Mood Swings—Now!* New York: Penguin.

Schachter, M. B. 2006. *What Your Doctor May Not Tell You About Depression: The Breakthrough Integrative Approach for Effective Treatment.* New York: Wellness Central.

Food, Cooking, and Cookbooks

Bennett, C. 2007. *Sugar Shock.* New York: Penguin Books.

Child, J. 2009. *Julia's Kitchen Wisdom.* New York: Random House.

Fallon, S., with M. Enig. 2001. *Nourishing Traditions: The Cookbook That Challenges Politically Correct Nutrition and the Diet Dictocrats.* Washington, DC: NewTrends Publishing.

Gittleman, A. L. 1996. *Get the Sugar Out.* New York: Random House.

Harvard School of Public Health. 2009. How sweet is it? See how much sugar is in soda, juice, sports drinks, and energy drinks. www.hsph.harvard.edu/nutritionsource/healthy-drinks/how-sweet-is-it/index.html.

Kirchner, B. 1995. *The Bold Vegetarian: 150 Innovative International Recipes.* New York: Harper Collins.

Matthews, J. 2010. *Cooking to Heal: Nutrition and Cooking Class for Autism.* San Francisco: Healthful Living Media.

Wood, R. 1999. *The New Whole Foods Encyclopedia.* New York: Penguin.

References

Abbey, L. C. 1982. Agoraphobia. *Journal of Orthomolecular Psychiatry* 11(4):243-259.

Adams, P. F., G. E. Hendershot, and M. A. Marano. 1999. Current estimates from the National Health Interview Survey 1996. *Vital Health Statistics* Series 10, 200:1-203.

Addolorato, G., D. di Giuda, G. de Rossi, et al. 2004. Regional cerebral hypoperfusion in patients with celiac disease. *American Journal of Medicine* 116(5):312-317.

Addolorato, G., A. Mirijello, C. D'Angelo, L. Leggio, A. Ferrulli, L. Abenavoli, et al. 2008. State and trait anxiety and depression in patients affected by gastrointestinal diseases: Psychometric evaluation of 1641 patients referred to an internal medicine outpatient setting. *International Journal of Clinical Practice* 62(7):1063-1069.

Addolorato, G., A. Mirijello, C. D'Angelo, L. Leggio, A. Ferrulli, L. Vonghia, et al. 2008. Social phobia in coeliac disease. *Scandinavian Journal of Gastroenterology* 43(4):410-415.

Akbaraly, T. N., E. J. Brunner, J. E. Ferrie, M. G. Marmot, M. Kivimaki, and A. Singh-Manoux. 2009. Dietary pattern and depressive symptoms in middle age. *British Journal of Psychiatry* 195(5):408-413.

Alarcón de la Lastra, C., M. D. Barranco, V. Motilva, and J. M. Herrerías. 2001. Mediterranean diet and health: Biological importance of olive oil. *Current Pharmaceutical Design* 7(10):933-950.

Alexander, D. D., and C. A. Cushing. 2010. Red meat and colorectal cancer: A critical summary of prospective epidemiologic studies. *Obesity*

Reviews, epub ahead of print, July 21. doi: 10.1111/j.1467-789X.2010. 00785.x

Amarasiri, W. A., and A. S. Dissanayake. 2006. Coconut fats. *Ceylon Medical Journal* 51(2):47-51.

Anderson, R. A., M. M. Polansky, N. A. Bryden, S. J. Bhathena, and J. J. Canary. 1987. Effects of supplemental chromium on patients with symptoms of reactive hypoglycemia. *Metabolism* 36(4):351-355.

Andrews, G., W. Hall, M. Teesson, and S. Henderson. 1999. *The Mental Health of Australians*. Canberra, Australia: Mental Health Branch, Commonwealth Department of Health and Aged Care.

Anxiety Disorders Association of America. 2010. Facts and Statistics. www .adaa.org/about-adaa/press-room/facts-statistics (accessed December 14, 2010).

Apóstolo, J. L., and K. Kolcaba. 2009. The effects of guided imagery on comfort, depression, anxiety, and stress of psychiatric inpatients with depressive disorders. *Archives of Psychiatric Nursing* 23(6):403-411.

Armstrong, D. J., G. K. Meenagh, I. Bickle, A. S. Lee, E. S. Curran, and M. B. Finch. 2007. Vitamin D deficiency is common in fibromyalgia and occurs more frequently in patients with anxiety and depression. *Clinical Rheumatology* 26(4):551-554.

Atkinson, W., T. A. Sheldon, N. Shaath, and P. J. Whorwell. 2004. Food elimination based on IgG antibodies in irritable bowel syndrome: A randomised controlled trial. *Gut* 53(10):1459-1464.

Austin G. L., C. B. Dalton, Y. Hu, et al. 2009. Diarrhea-predominant irritable bowel syndrome. *Clinical Gastroenterology and Hepatology* 7(6):706-708.

Avants, S. K., and A. Margolin. 1995. "Self" and addiction: The role of imagery in self-regulation. *Journal of Alternative and Complementary Medicine* 1(4):339-345.

Badawy, A. A. 2003. Alcohol and violence and the possible role of sero-tonin. *Criminal Behaviour and Mental Health* 13(1):31-44.

Baines, S., J. Powers, and W. J. Brown. 2007. How does the health and well-being of young Australian vegetarian and semi-vegetarian women compare with non-vegetarians? *Public Health Nutrition* 10(5):436-442.

Banderet, L. E., and H. R. Lieberman. 1989. Treatment with tyrosine, a neurotransmitter precursor, reduces environmental stress in humans. *Brain Research Bulletin* 22(4):759-762.

Barker, J. M., and E. Liu. 2008. Celiac disease: Pathophysiology, clinical manifestations, and associated autoimmune conditions. *Advances in Pediatrics* 55:349-365.

Benor, D. J., K. Ledger, L. Toussaint, G. Hett, and D. Zaccaro. 2009. Pilot study of emotional freedom techniques, wholistic hybrid derived from eye movement desensitization and reprocessing and emotional freedom technique, and cognitive behavioral therapy for treatment of test anxiety in university students. *Explore* (NY) 5(6):338-340.

Benton, D., and R. T. Donohoe. 1999. The effects of nutrients on mood. *Public Health Nutrition* 2(3A):403-409.

Birdsall, T. C. 1998. 5-Hydroxytryptophan: A clinically-effective serotonin precursor. *Alternative Medicine Review* 3(4):271-280.

Blaylock, R. L. 1997. *Excitotoxins: The Taste That Kills.* Santa Fe, NM: Health Press.

Blum, K., E. R. Braverman, J. M. Holder, et al. 2000. Reward deficiency syndrome: A biogenetic model for the diagnosis and treatment of impulsive, addictive, and compulsive behaviors. *Journal of Psychoactive Drugs* 32(Suppl):i-iv, 1-112.

Bolin, T. 2009. IBS or intolerance? *Australian Family Physician* 38(12):962-965.

Bouchard, M. F., D. C. Bellinger, J. Weuve, et al. 2009. Blood lead levels and major depressive disorder, panic disorder, and generalized anxiety disorder in U.S. young adults. *Archives of General Psychiatry* 66(12):1313-1319.

Bouchard, M. F., D. C. Bellinger, R. O. Wright, and M. G. Weisskopf. 2010. Attention-deficit/hyperactivity disorder and urinary metabolites of organophosphate pesticides. *Pediatrics* 125(6):e1270-1277. doi: 10.1542/peds.2009-3058.

Bourne, E. J., A. Brownstein, and L. Garano. 2004. *Natural Relief for Anxiety: Complementary Strategies for Easing Fear, Panic, and Worry.* Oakland, CA: New Harbinger Publications.

Bradstock, M. K., M. K. Serdula, J. S. Marks, et al. 1986. Evaluation of reactions to food additives: The aspartame experience. *American Journal of Clinical Nutrition* 43(3):464-469.

Braly, J., and R. Hoggan. 2002. *Dangerous Grains: Why Gluten Cereal Grains May Be Hazardous to Your Health.* New York: Penguin Putnam.

Braverman, E. R. 2003. *The Healing Nutrients Within.* Laguna Beach, CA: Basic Health Publications.

Braverman, E. R., and E. Weissberg. 1987. Elevated IgE levels in patients with low whole blood histamine. *Journal of Orthomolecular Medicine* 2(4):219-220.

Brody, S., R. Preut, K. Schommer, and T. H. Schürmeyer. 2002. A randomized controlled trial of high dose ascorbic acid for reduction of blood pressure, cortisol, and subjective responses to psychological stress. *Psychopharmacology* 159(3):319-324.

Brown, M. J., M. G. Ferruzzi, M. L. Nguyen, et al. 2004. Carotenoid bio-availability is higher from salads ingested with full fat than with fat-reduced salad dressings as measured with electrochemical detection. *American Journal of Clinical Nutrition* 80(2):396-403.

Brown, R. P., and P. L. Gerbarg. 2005. Yogic breathing in the treatment of stress, anxiety, and depression: Part II—clinical applications and guidelines. *Journal of Alternative and Complementary Medicine* 11(4):711-717.

Bruce, M. S., and M. Lader. 1989. Caffeine abstention in the management of anxiety disorders. *Psychological Medicine* 19(1):211-214.

Bujatti, M., and P. Riederer. 1976. Serotonin, noradrenaline, dopamine metabolites in transcendental meditation technique. *Journal of Neural Transmission* 39(3):257-267.

Burt, C. W., and S. M. Schappert. 2004. Ambulatory care visits to physician offices, hospital outpatient departments, and emergency departments: United States 1999-2000. *Vital Health Statistics* Series 13, 157:1-70.

Buydens-Branchey, L., M. Branchey, and J. R. Hibbeln. 2008. Associations between increases in plasma n-3 polyunsaturated fatty acids following supplementation and decreases in anger and anxiety in substance abusers. *Progress in Neuro-Psychopharmacology and Biological Psychiatry* 32(2):568-575.

Campbell-McBride, N. 2008. *Gut and Psychology Syndrome: Natural Treatment for Autism, ADD/ADHD, Dyslexia, Dyspraxia, Depression, Schizophrenia.* Cambridge, UK: Medinform Publishing.

Cannell, J. 2010. Vitamin D Council Statement on FNB Vitamin D Report. www.vitamindcouncil.org/vdc-statement-fnb-vitamin-d-report.shtml (accessed December 18, 2010).

Cassels, C. 2010. Whole diet may ward off depression and anxiety. *Medscape Medical News.* www.medscape.com/viewarticle/715239 (accessed December 17, 2010).

Cater, R. E. 1992. The clinical importance of hypochlorhydria (a consequence of chronic *Helicobacter* infection): Its possible etiological role in mineral and amino acid malabsorption, depression, and other syndromes. *Medical Hypotheses* 39(4):375-383.

Celec, P., and M. Behuliak. 2010. Behavioural and endocrine effects of chronic cola intake. *Journal of Psychopharmacology* 24(10):1569-1572.

Charney, D. S., G. R. Heninger, and P. I. Jatlow. 1985. Increased anxiogenic effects of caffeine in panic disorders. *Archives of General Psychiatry* 42(3):233-243.

Child, J. 2009. *Julia's Kitchen Wisdom.* New York: Random House.

Cho, H. S., S. Kim, S. Y. Lee, J. A. Park, S. J. Kim, and H. S. Chun. 2008. Protective effect of the green tea component, L-theanine on environmental toxins–induced neuronal cell death. *Neurotoxicology* 29(4):656-662.

Clementz, G. L., and J. W. Dailey. 1988. Psychotropic effects of caffeine. *American Family Physician* 37(5):167-172.

Cordain, L. S. 2001. *The Paleo Diet: Lose Weight and Get Healthy by Eating the Food You Were Designed to Eat.* Hoboken, NJ: Wiley.

Corrao, G., G. R. Corazza, V. Bagnardi, et al. 2001. Mortality in patients with coeliac disease and their relatives: A cohort study. *Lancet* 358(9279):356-361.

Corti, R., J. Perdrix, A. J. Flammer, and G. Noll G. 2010. Dark or white chocolate? Cocoa and cardiovascular health. *Revue Medical Suisse* 6(239):499-500, 502-504.

Corwin, R. L., and P. S. Grigson. 2009. Symposium overview. Food addiction: Fact or fiction? *Journal of Nutrition* 139(3):617-619.

Crook, W. G. 1997. *The Yeast Connection and the Woman.* Jackson, TN: Professional Books.

Dadd, D. L. 1997. *Home Safe Home: Protecting Yourself and Your Family from Everyday Toxics and Harmful Household Products.* New York: Jeremy P. Tarcher/Penguin.

Daley, C. A., A. Abbott, P. S. Doyle, G. A. Nader, and S. Larson. 2010. A review of fatty acid profiles and antioxidant content in grass-fed and grain-fed beef. *Nutrition Journal* 9:10.

Daniel, K. T. 2003. Why broth is beautiful: Essential roles for proline, glycine, and gelatin. *Wise Traditions in Food, Farming, and the Healing Arts*, Spring, 25-36. westonaprice.org/food-features/513-why-broth-is-beautiful.html (Acessed December 16, 2010).

Darlington, L., N. W. Ramsey, and J. R. Mansfield. 1986. Placebo-controlled, blind study of dietary manipulation therapy in rheumatoid arthritis. *Lancet* 1(8475):236-238.

Davidson, J. R., K. Abraham, K. M. Connor, and M. N. McLeod. 2003. Effectiveness of chromium in atypical depression: A placebo-controlled trial. *Biological Psychiatry* 53(3):261-264.

Davis, D. R. 2009. Declining fruit and vegetable nutrient composition: What is the evidence? *HortScience* 44:15-19.

de Bloom, J., M. Kompier, S. Geurts, C. de Weerth, T. Taris, and S. Sonnentag. 2009. Do we recover from vacation? Meta-analysis of vacation effects on health and well-being. *Journal of Occupational Health* 51(1):13-25.

de Souza, M. C., A. F. Walker, P. A. Robinson, and K. Bolland. 2000. A synergistic effect of a daily supplement for 1 month of 200 mg magnesium plus 50 mg vitamin B_6 for the relief of anxiety-related premenstrual symptoms: A randomized, double-blind, crossover study. *Journal of Women's Health and Gender-Based Medicine* 9(2):131-139.

de Vendômois, J. S., D. Cellier, C. Vélot, E. Clair, R. Mesnage, and G. E. Séralini. 2010. Debate on GMO's health risks after statistical findings in regulatory tests. *International Journal of Biological Sciences* 6(6):590-598.

di Cagno, R., M. de Angelis, S. Auricchio, et al. 2004. Sourdough bread made from wheat and nontoxic flours and started with selected lactobacilli is tolerated in celiac sprue patients. *Applied and Environmental Microbiology* 70(2):1088-1096.

Druss, B. G., and R. A. Rosenheck. 2000. Use of practitioner-based complementary therapies by persons reporting mental conditions in the United States. *Archives of General Psychiatry* 57(7):708-714.

Du, D., Y. H. Shi, and G. W. Le. 2010. Microarray analysis of high-glucose diet-induced changes in mRNA expression in jejunums of C57BL/6J mice reveals impairment in digestion, absorption. *Molecular Biology Reports* 37(4):1867-1874.

Dufault, R., B. LeBlanc, R. Schnoll, et al. 2009. Mercury from chlor-alkali plants: Measured concentrations in food product sugar. *Environmental Health* 8:2.

Duntas, L. H. 2009. Does celiac disease trigger autoimmune thyroiditis? *Nature Reviews. Endocrinology* 5(4):190-191.

Edelman, E. 2001. *Natural Healing for Schizophrenia and Other Common Mental Disorders*. Eugene, OR: Borage Books.

Environmental Working Group. 2010. EWG's Shopper's Guide to Pesticides. http://static.foodnews.org/pdf/EWG-shoppers-guide.pdf (accessed December 9, 2010).

Fallon, S. 2001. *Nourishing Traditions: The Cookbook That Challenges Politically Correct Nutrition and the Diet Dictocrats*. With M. Enig. Washington, DC: NewTrends Publishing.

Feldman, M., and C. T. Richardson. 1986. Role of thought, sight, smell, and taste of food in the cephalic phase of gastric acid secretion in humans. *Gastroenterology* 90(2):428-433.

Fernstrom, J. D. 1981. Effects of the diet on brain function. *Acta Astronautica* 8(9-10):1035-1042.

Freeman, M. P. 2010. Nutrition and psychiatry. *American Journal of Psychiatry* 167(3):244-247.

Gaby, A. R. 2004. Recurrent candidiasis: One step forward, still backward. Editorial. *Townsend Letter*, November. townsendletter.com/Nov2004/gabyeditorial1104.htm (accessed December 6, 2010).

Galland, L. 1985. Nutrition and candidiasis. *Journal of Orthomolecular Medicine* 14(1):50-60.

Gershon, M. 1998. *The Second Brain: A Groundbreaking New Understanding of Nervous Disorders of the Stomach and Intestine.* New York: Harper Collins.

Gittleman, A. L. 1998. *Before the Change: Taking Charge of Your Perimenopause.* San Francisco: Harper Collins.

Goodwin, R. D., P. M. Lewinsohn, and J. R. Seeley. 2005. Cigarette smoking and panic attacks among young adults in the community: The role of parental smoking and anxiety disorders. *Biological Psychiatry* 58(9):686-693.

Gottschall, E. G. 2002. *Breaking the Vicious Cycle: Intestinal Health Through Diet.* Baltimore, Ontario, Canada: Kirkton Press.

Greden, J. F. 1974. Anxiety or caffeinism: A diagnostic dilemma. *American Journal of Psychiatry* 131(10):1089-1092.

Haag, M. 2003. Essential fatty acids and the brain. *Canadian Journal of Psychiatry* 48(3):195-203.

Hallert, C., M. Svensson, J. Tholstrup, and B. Hultberg. 2009. Clinical trial: B vitamins improve health in coeliac patients living on a gluten-free diet. *Alimentary Pharmacology and Therapeutics* 29(8):811-816.

Hamer, H. M., D. Jonkers, K. Venema, S. Vanhoutvin, F. J. Troost, and R. J. Brummer. 2008. Review article: The role of butyrate on colonic function. *Alimentary Pharmacology and Therapeutics* 27(2):104-119.

Harp, M. J., and L. W. Fox. 1990. Correlations of the physical symptoms of hypoglycemia with the psychological symptoms of anxiety and depression. *Journal of Orthomolecular Medicine* 5(1):8-10.

Harvard School of Public Health. 2009. How sweet is it? See how much sugar is in soda, juice, sports drinks, and energy drinks. www.hsph.harvard.edu/nutritionsource/healthy-drinks/how-sweet-is-it/index.html (accessed December 10, 2010).

Hausch, F., L. Shan, N. A. Santiago, G. M. Gray, and C. Khosla. 2002. Intestinal digestive resistance of immunodominant gliadin peptides. *American Journal of Physiology* Gastrointestinal and Liver Physiology 283(4):G996-1003.

Hawrelak, J. A., and S. P. Myers. 2004. The causes of intestinal dysbiosis: A review. *Alternative Medical Review* 9(2):180-197.

Head, K. A., and G. S. Kelly. 2009. Nutrients and botanicals for treatment of stress: Adrenal fatigue, neurotransmitter imbalance, anxiety, and restless sleep. *Alternative Medicine Review* 14(2):114-140.

Heleniak, E. P., and S. W. Lamola. 1986. A new prostaglandin disturbance syndrome in schizophrenia: Delta-6-pyroluria. *Medical Hypotheses* 19(4):333-338.

Heseker, H., W. Kübler, V. Pudel, and J. Westenhöffer. 1992. Psychological disorders as early symptoms of a mild-to-moderate vitamin deficiency. *Annals of the New York Academy of Sciences* 669:352-357.

Hoehn-Saric, R. 1982. Neurotransmitters in anxiety. *Archives of General Psychiatry* 39(6):735-742.

Hoffer, A. 1995. The discovery of kryptopyrrole and its importance in diagnosis of biochemical imbalances in schizophrenia and in criminal behavior. *Journal of Orthomolecular Medicine* 10(1):3-7.

Hoffer, A., and M. Walker. 1996. *Putting It All Together: The New Orthomolecular Nutrition.* New Canaan, CT: Keats Publishing.

Hudson, C., S. Hudson, and J. MacKenzie. 2007. Protein-source tryptophan as an efficacious treatment for social anxiety disorder: A pilot study. *Canadian Journal of Physiological Pharmacology* 85(9):928-932.

Hulley, S. B., J. M. Walsh, and T. B. Newman. 1992. Health policy on blood cholesterol: Time to change directions. *Circulation* 86(3):1026-1029.

Humphries, P., E. Pretorius, and H. Naudé. 2008. Direct and indirect cellular effects of aspartame on the brain. *European Journal of Clinical Nutrition* 62(4):451-462.

Hyman, M. 2009. *The UltraMind Solution: Fixing Your Broken Brain by Healing Your Body First.* New York: Simon and Schuster.

Ifland, J. R., H. G. Preuss, M. T. Marcus, et al. 2009. Refined food addiction: A classic substance use disorder. *Medical Hypotheses* 72(5):518-526.

Jacka, F. N., J. A. Pasco, A. Mykletun, L. J. Williams, A. M. Hodge, et al. 2010. Association of Western and traditional diets with depression and anxiety in women. *American Journal of Psychiatry* 167(3):305-311.

Jacka, F. N., J. A. Pasco, A. Mykletun, L. J. Williams, G. C. Nicholson, et al. 2010. Diet quality in bipolar disorder in a population-based sample of women. *Journal of Affective Disorders*, epub ahead of print, September 30. doi: 10.1016/j.jad.2010.09.004.

Jackson, J. A., H. D. Riordan, R. Hunninghake, and C. Revard. 1999. *Candida albicans*: The hidden infection. *Journal of Orthomolecular Medicine* 14(4):198-200.

Jackson, J. A., H. D. Riordan, S. Neathery, and C. Revard. 1998. Histamine levels in health and diseases. *Journal of Orthomolecular Medicine* 13(4):236-240.

Jacobs, G. 1997. *Beat Candida Through Diet.* London: Random House.

Johnson, R. K., L. J. Appel, M. Brands, et al. 2009. Dietary sugars intake and cardiovascular health: A scientific statement from the American Heart Association. *Circulation* 120(11):1011-1020.

Jolanda, M., R. A. Verheij, S. de Vries, P. Spreeuwenberg, F. G. Schellevis, and P. P. Groenewegen. 2009. Morbidity is related to a green living environment. *Journal of Epidemiology and Community Health* 63(12):967-973.

Jones, P. J. 2009. Dietary cholesterol and the risk of cardiovascular disease in patients: A review of the Harvard Egg Study and other data. *International Journal of Clinical Practice* Supplement 163:1-8, 28-36.

Juliano, L. M., and R. R. Griffiths. 2004. A critical review of caffeine withdrawal: Empirical validation of symptoms and signs, incidence, severity, and associated features. *Psychopharmacology* 176(1):1-29.

Kahn, R. S., H. G. Westenberg, W. Verhoeven, et al. 1987. Effect of a serotonin precursor and uptake inhibitor in anxiety disorders: A double-blind comparison of 5-hydroxytryptophan, clomipramin, and placebo. *International Clinical Psychopharmacology* 2(1):33-45.

Kalaydjian, A. E., W. Eaton, N. Cascella, and A. Fasano. 2006. The gluten connection: The association between schizophrenia and celiac disease. *Acta Psychiatrica Scandinavica* 113(2):82-90.

Kessler, R. C., J. Soukup, R. B. Davis, et al. 2001. The use of complementary and alternative therapies to treat anxiety and depression in the United States. *American Journal of Psychiatry* 158(2):289-294.

Ketcham, K., and L. A. Mueller. 1983. *Eating Right to Live Sober.* Seattle: Madrona Publishers.

Kidd, R. F. 2000. Results of dental amalgam removal and mercury detoxification using DMPS and neural therapy. *Alternative Therapies in Health and Medicine* 6(4):49-55.

Kim, J. H., D. Desor, Y. T. Kim, et al. 2007. Efficacy of alphas1-casein hydrolysate on stress-related symptoms in women. *European Journal of Clinical Nutrition* 61(4):536-541.

Kimura, K., M. Ozeki, L. R. Juneja, and H. Ohira. 2007. L-theanine reduces psychological and physiological stress responses. *Biological Psychology* 74(1):39-45.

King, D. S. 1984. Psychological and behavioral effects of food and chemical exposure in sensitive individuals. *Nutrition and Health* 3(3):137-151.

King, T. S., M. Elia, and J. O. Hunter. 1998. Abnormal colonic fermentation in irritable bowel syndrome. *Lancet* 352:1187–1189.

Kirchner, B. 1995. *The Bold Vegetarian: 150 Innovative International Recipes.* New York: Harper Collins.

Kolahdooz, F., J. C. van der Pols, C. J. Bain, et al. 2010. Meat, fish, and ovarian cancer risk: Results from 2 Australian case-control studies, a systematic review, and meta-analysis. *American Journal of Clinical Nutrition* 91(6):1752-1763.

Lajous, M., M. C. Boutron-Ruault, A. Fabre, F. Clavel-Chapelon, and I. Romieu. 2008. Carbohydrate intake, glycemic index, glycemic load, and risk of postmenopausal breast cancer in a prospective study of French women. *American Journal of Clinical Nutrition* 87(5):1384-1391.

Lake, J. 2007. *Textbook of Integrative Mental Health.* New York: Thieme Medical.

Lansdowne, A. T., and S. C. Provost. 1998. Vitamin D_3 enhances mood in healthy subjects during winter. *Psychopharmacology* 135(4):319-323.

Lara, D. R. 2010. Caffeine, mental health, and psychiatric disorders. *Journal of Alzheimer's Disease* 20(Suppl. 1):S239-248.

Lehnert, H., and R. J. Wurtman. 1993. Amino acid control of neurotransmitter synthesis and release: Physiological and clinical implications. *Psychotherapy and Psychosomatics* 60(1):18-32.

Levi, L. 1967. The effect of coffee on the function of the sympatho-adreno-medullary system in man. *Acta Medica Scandinavica* 181(4):431-438.

Lewis, S. J., and K. W. Heaton. 1997. Stool form scale as a useful guide to intestinal transit time. *Scandinavian Journal of Gastroenterology* 32(9):920-924.

Lipski, E. 2004. *Digestive Wellness.* New York: McGraw Hill.

Lord, R. S., and J. A. Bralley (eds.). 2008. *Laboratory Evaluations for Integrative and Functional Medicine.* Duluth, GA: Metametrix Institute.

Lydiard, R. B. 2001. Irritable bowel syndrome, anxiety, and depression: What are the links? *Journal of Clinical Psychiatry* 62(Suppl. 8):38-45; discussion 46-47.

———. 2003. The role of GABA in anxiety disorders. *Journal of Clinical Psychiatry* 64(3):21-27.

Macht, M., and D. Dettmer. 2006. Everyday mood and emotions after eating a chocolate bar or an apple. *Appetite* 46(3):332-336.

Maddock, R. J., C. S. Carter, and D. W. Gietzen. 1991. Elevated serum lactate associated with panic attacks induced by hyperventilation. *Psychiatry Research* 38(3):301-311.

Maron, E., I. Toru, V. Vasar, and J. Shlik. 2004. The effect of 5-hydroxy-tryptophan on cholecystokinin-4-induced panic attacks in healthy volunteers. *Journal of Psychopharmacology* 18(2):194-199.

Marriott, P. F., K. M. Greenwood, and S. M. Armstrong. 1994. Seasonality in panic disorder. *Journal of Affective Disorders* 31(2):75-80.

Maskarinec, G. 2009. Cancer protective properties of cocoa: A review of the epidemiologic evidence. *Nutrition and Cancer* 61(5):573-579.

Mathews-Larson, J. 2001. *Depression-Free Naturally: 7 Weeks to Eliminating Anxiety, Despair, Fatigue, and Anger from Your Life.* New York: Random House.

McCarty, M. 2000. High-dose pyridoxine as an "anti-stress" strategy. *Medical Hypotheses* 54(5):803-807.

McGinnis, W. R., T. Audhya, W. J. Walsh, et al. 2008a. Discerning the mauve factor, part 1. *Alternative Therapies in Health and Medicine* 14(2):40-50.

———. 2008b. Discerning the mauve factor, part 2. *Alternative Therapies in Health and Medicine* 14(3):56-62.

McKenna, S. 2002. *The Phytogenic Hormone Solution.* New York: Random House.

Mearns, J., J. Dunn, and P. R. Lees-Haley. 1994. Psychological effects of organophosphate pesticides: A review and call for research by psychologists. *Journal of Clinical Psychology* 50(2):286-294.

Mebane, A. H. 1984. L-glutamine and mania. *American Journal of Psychiatry* 141(10):1302-1303.

MedlinePlus. 2009. Caffeine in the diet. www.nlm.nih.gov/medlineplus/ency/article/002445.htm (accessed December 6, 2010).

Micha, R., S. K. Wallace, and D. Mozaffarian. 2010. Red and processed meat consumption and risk of incident coronary heart disease, stroke, and diabetes mellitus: A systematic review and meta-analysis. *Circulation* 121(21):2271-2283.

Miller, A. L. 1999. Therapeutic considerations of L-glutamine: A review of the literature. *Alternative Medicine Review* 4(4):239-248.

Möhler, H., P. Polc, R. Cumin, L. Pieri, and R. Kettler. 1979. Nicotinamide is a brain constituent with benzodiazepine-like actions. *Nature* 278(5704):563-565.

Monteiro, M. G., M. A. Schuckit, and M. Irwin. 1990. Subjective feelings of anxiety in young men after ethanol and diazepam infusions. *Journal of Clinical Psychiatry* 51(1):12-16.

Mulligan, G. B., and A. Licata. 2010. Taking vitamin D with the largest meal improves absorption and results in higher serum levels of 25-hydroxyvitamin D. *Journal of Bone and Mineral Research* 25(4):928-930.

Murooka, Y., and M. Yamshita. 2008. Traditional healthful fermented products of Japan. *Journal of Industrial Microbiology and Biotechnology* 35(8):791-798.

Murray, M. T., and J. E. Pizzorno. 1998. *Encyclopedia of Natural Medicine.* Roseville, CA: Prima Publishing.

Naiyer, A. J., J. Shah, L. Hernandez, et al. 2008. Tissue transglutaminase antibodies in individuals with celiac disease bind to thyroid follicles and extracellular matrix and may contribute to thyroid dysfunction. *Thyroid* 18(11):1171-1178.

Nathan, R. A. 2007. The burden of allergic rhinitis. *Allergy and Asthma Proceedings* 28(1):3-9.

National Coffee Association. 2009. *2009 National Coffee Drinking Trends.* New York: National Coffee Association. Statistics cited in an online press release, available at www.ncausa.org/custom/headlines/headline-details.cfm?id=691&returnto=171. Accessed December 15, 2010.

National Sleep Foundation. 2009. 2009 Health and Safety Sleep in America Polls. www.sleepfoundation.org/article/sleep-america-polls/2009-health-and-safety (accessed December 17, 2010).

Nutt, D. J. 2001. Neurobiological mechanisms in generalized anxiety disorder. *Journal of Clinical Psychiatry* 62(Suppl 11):22-27; discussion 28.

O'Carroll, R. E., G. Masterton, N. Dougall, K. P. Ebmeier, and G. M. Goodwin. 1995. The neuropsychiatric sequelae of mercury poisoning: The Mad Hatter's disease revisited. *British Journal of Psychiatry* 167(1):95-98.

Palatnik, A., K. Frolov, M. Fux, and J. Benjamin. 2001. Double-blind, controlled, crossover trial of inositol versus fluvoxamine for the treatment of panic disorder. *Journal of Clinical Psychopharmacology* 21(3):335-339.

Pelton, R., J. B. LaValle, and E. B. Hawkins. 2001. *Drug-Induced Nutrient Depletion Handbook.* Hudson, OH: Lexi-Comp.

Perez-Rodriguez, M. M., E. Baca-Garcia, C. Diaz-Sastre, et al. 2008. Low serum cholesterol may be associated with suicide attempt history. *Journal of Clinical Psychiatry* 69(12):1920-1927.

Petruzzello, S. J., D. M. Landers, B. D. Hatfield, K. A. Kubitz, and W. D. Salazar. 1991. A meta-analysis on the anxiety-reducing effects of acute and chronic exercise. *Sports Medicine* 11(3):143-182.

Pfeiffer, C. 1987. *Nutrition and Mental Illness.* Rochester, VT: Healing Arts Press.

Pfeiffer, C., A. Sohler, C. H. Jenney, and V. Iliev. 1974. Treatment of pyroluric schizophrenia (malvaria) with large doses of pyridoxine and a dietary supplement of zinc. *Journal of Orthomolecular Psychiatry* 3(4):292-300.

Pilkington, K., G. Kirkwood, H. Rampes, M. Cummings, and J. Richardson. 2007. Acupuncture for anxiety and anxiety disorders: A systematic literature review. *Acupuncture in Medicine* 25(1-2):1-10.

Pitozzi, V., M. Jacomelli, M. Zaid, et al. 2010. Effects of dietary extra-virgin olive oil on behaviour and brain biochemical parameters in ageing rats. *British Journal of Nutrition* 103(11):1674-1683.

Pizzorno, J. E., and M. T. Murray. 2000. *Textbook of Natural Medicine*. London: Harcourt.

Potocki, P., and K. Hozyasz. 2002. Psychiatric symptoms and coeliac disease [article in Polish]. *Psychiatria Polska* 36(4):567-578.

Prasad, A. S. 1985. Clinical manifestations of zinc deficiency. *Annual Revue of Nutrition* 5:341-363.

Preis, S. R., M. J. Stampfer, D. Spiegelman, W. C. Willett, and E. B. Rimm. 2010. Lack of association between dietary protein intake and risk of stroke among middle-aged men. *American Journal of Clinical Nutrition* 91(1):39-45.

Prousky, J. E. 2004. Niacinamide's potential role in alleviating anxiety with its benzodiazepine-like properties: A case report. *Journal of Orthomolecular Medicine* 19(2):104-110.

——. 2006. *Anxiety: Orthomolecular Diagnosis and Treatment*. Ottawa, Ontario, Canada: CCNM Press.

Pynnönen, P., E. Isometsä, E. Aronen, M. Verkasalo, E. Savilahti, and V. Aalberg. 2004. Mental disorders in adolescents with celiac disease. *Psychosomatics* 45:325-335.

Pynnönen, P., E. Isometsä, M. Verkasalo, et al. 2005. Gluten-free diet may alleviate depressive and behavioural symptoms in adolescents with coeliac disease: A prospective follow-up case-series study. *BMC Psychiatry* 5:14.

Ralston, N. V., and L. J. Raymond. 2010. Dietary selenium's protective effects against methylmercury toxicity. *Toxicology* 278(1):112-123.

Ramsden, C. E., K. R. Faurot, P. Carrera-Bastos, L. S. Sperling, M. de Lorgeril, and L. Cordain. 2009. Dietary fat quality and coronary heart disease prevention: A unified theory based on evolutionary, historical, global, and modern perspectives. *Current Treatment Options in Cardiovascular Medicine* 11(4):289-301.

Rao, A. V., A. C. Bested, T. M. Beaulne, et al. 2009. A randomized, double-blind, placebo-controlled pilot study of a probiotic in emotional symptoms of chronic fatigue syndrome. *Gut Pathogens* 1(1):6.

Rho, K. H., S. H. Han, K. S. Kim, and M. S. Lee. 2006. Effects of aroma-therapy massage on anxiety and self-esteem in Korean elderly women: A pilot study. *International Journal of Neuroscience* 116(12):1447-1455.

Rippere, V. 1984. Some varieties of food intolerance in psychiatric patients: An overview. *Nutrition and Health* 3(3):125-136.

Rogers, C. E., L. K. Larkey, and C. Keller. 2009. A review of clinical trials of tai chi and qigong in older adults. *Western Journal of Nursing Research* 31(2):245-279.

Ross, J. 2004. *The Mood Cure: The 4-Step Program to Take Charge of Your Emotions—Today.* New York: Penguin.

———. 2006. Urinary neurotransmitter testing: Problems and alternatives. *Townsend Letter,* October. www.dietcure.com/urinetesting.pdf (accessed December 27, 2010).

———. 2011. *The Diet Cure: The 8-Step Program to Rebalance Your Body Chemistry, End Food Cravings, Weight Problems, and Mood Swings— Now!* New York: Penguin

Ruxton, C. 2010. Recommendations for the use of eggs in the diet. *Nursing Standard* 24(37):47-55.

Ruzzin, J., R. Petersen, E. Meugnier, et al. 2010. Persistent organic pollutant exposure leads to insulin resistance syndrome. *Environmental Health Perspectives* 118(4):465-471.

Sanchez, A., J. L. Reeser, H. S. Lau, et al. 1973. Role of sugars in human neutrophilic phagocytosis. *American Journal of Clinical Nutrition* 261(11):1180-1184.

Sanchez-Villegas, A., L. Verberne, J. De Irala, et al. 2011. Dietary fat intake and the risk of depression: The SUN Project. *PLoS One* 6(1):e16268.

Sanchez-Villegas, A., M. Delgado-Rodriguez, A. Alonso, et al. 2009. Association of the Mediterranean dietary pattern with the incidence of depression. *Archives of General Psychiatry* 66(10):1090-1098.

Schmidt, M. H., P. Möcks, B. Lay, et al. 1997. Does oligoantigenic diet influence hyperactive/conduct-disordered children: A controlled trial. *European Child and Adolescent Psychiatry* 6(2):88-95.

Schnoll, R., D. Burshteyn, and J. Cea-Aravena. 2003. Nutrition in the treatment of attention-deficit hyperactivity disorder: A neglected but important aspect. *Applied Psychophysiology and Biofeedback* 28(1):63-75.

Schwartz, T. L., N. Nihalani, S. Jindal, S. Virk, and N. Jones. 2004. Psychiatric medication–induced obesity: A review. *Obesity Reviews* 5(2):115-121.

Seelig, M. S. 1994. Consequences of magnesium deficiency on the enhancement of stress reactions: Preventive and therapeutic implications (a review). *Journal of the American College of Nutrition* 13(5):429-446.

Setzer, W. N. 2009. Essential oils and anxiolytic aromatherapy. *Natural Product Communications* 4(9):1305-1316.

Shakib, F., H. Morrow-Brown, A. Phelps, and R. Redhead. 2006. Study of IgG sub-class antibodies in patients with milk intolerance. *Clinical and Experimental Allergy* 16(5):451-458.

Shannahoff-Khalsa, D. S. 2004. An introduction to Kundalini yoga meditation techniques that are specific for the treatment of psychiatric disorders. *Journal of Alternative and Complementary Medicine* 10(1):91-101.

Silk, D. B., A. Davis, J. Vulevic, G. Tzortzis, and G. R. Gibson. 2009. Clinical trial: The effects of a trans-galactooligosaccharide prebiotic on faecal microbiota and symptoms in irritable bowel syndrome. *Alimentary Pharmacology and Therapeutics* 29(5):508-518.

Skaer, T. L., D. A. Sclar, and L. M. Robison. 2008. Trend in anxiety disorders in the USA 1990-2003. *Primary Care and Community Psychiatry* 13(1):1-7.

Smoller, J. W., M. H. Pollack, S. Wassertheil-Smoller, et al. 2007. Panic attacks and risk of incident cardiovascular events among postmenopausal women in the Women's Health Initiative Observational Study. *Archives of General Psychiatry* 64(10):1153-1160.

Stahl, L. A., D. P. Begg, R. S. Weisinger, and A. J. Sinclair. 2008. The role of omega-3 fatty acids in mood disorders. *Current Opinion in Investigational Drugs* 9(1):57-64.

Stanhope, K. L., and P. J. Havel. 2010. Fructose consumption: Recent results and their potential implications. *Annals of the New York Academy of Sciences* 1190(1):15-24.

Stiefel, F., and D. Stagno. 2004. Management of insomnia in patients with chronic pain conditions. *CNS Drugs* 18(5):285-296.

Stitt, B. 2002. *Impact of Fresh, Healthy Foods on Learning and Behavior* (DVD). Manitowoc, WI: Natural Press.

Strauss-Blasche, G., C. Ekmekcioglu, and W. Marktl. 2000. Does vacation enable recuperation? Changes in well-being associated with time away from work. *Occupational Medicine* 50(3):167-172.

Streeter, C. C., J. E. Jensen, R. M. Perlmutter, et al. 2007. Yoga asana sessions increase brain GABA levels: A pilot study. *Journal of Alternative and Complementary Medicine* 13(4):419-426.

Suarez, E. C. 1999. Relations of trait depression and anxiety to low lipid and lipoprotein concentrations in healthy young adult women. *Psychosomatic Medicine* 61(3):273-279.

Tanskanen, A., J. R. Hibbeln, J. Tuomilehto, et al. 2001. Fish consumption and depressive symptoms in the general population in Finland. *Psychiatric Services* 52(4):529-531.

Tkachuk, G. A., and G. L. Martin. 1999. Exercise therapy for patients with psychiatric disorders: Research and clinical implications. *Professional Psychology: Research and Practice* 30(3):275-282.

Tsaluchidu, S., M. Cocchi, L. Tonello, and B. K. Puri. 2008. Fatty acids and oxidative stress in psychiatric disorders. *BMC Psychiatry* 17(8, Suppl. 1):S5.

Uspenskii, I. P., and E. V. Balukova. 2009. Pathomorphosis of anxiety disorder in patients with intestinal dysbiosis [article in Russian]. [*Experimental and Clinical Gastroenterology*] 7:91-96.

Vally, H., and P. J. Thompson. 2003. Allergic and asthmatic reactions to alcoholic drinks. *Addiction Biology* 8(1):3-11.

van Mill, J. G., W. J. Hoogendijk, N. Vogelzangs, R. van Dyck, and B. W. Penninx. 2010. Insomnia and sleep duration in a large cohort of patients with major depressive disorder and anxiety disorders. *Journal of Clinical Psychiatry* 71(3):239-246.

Wallwork, J. C. 1987. Zinc and the central nervous system. *Progress in Food and Nutrition Science* 11(2):203-247.

Walsh, W. J. 1991. Biochemical treatment: Medicines for the next century. *NOHA News* 16(3):2-4.

Walters, K., G. Rait, I. Petersen, R. Williams, and I. Nazareth. 2008. Panic disorder and risk of new onset coronary heart disease, acute myocardial infarction, and cardiac mortality: Cohort study using the general practice research database. *European Heart Journal* 29(24):2981-2988.

Wells, A. S., N. W. Read, J. D. Laugharne, and N. S. Ahluwalia. 1998. Alterations in mood after changing to a low-fat diet. *British Journal of Nutrition* 79(1):23-30.

Werbach, M. R. 1999. *Nutritional Influences on Mental Illness*. Tarzana, CA: Third Line Press.

West, R., and P. Hajek. 1997. What happens to anxiety levels on giving up smoking? *American Journal of Psychiatry* 154(11):1589-1592.

Westen, D., and K. A. Morrison. 2001. A multidimensional meta-analysis of treatments for depression, panic, and generalized anxiety disorder: An empirical examination of the status of empirically supported therapies. *Journal of Consulting and Clinical Psychology* 69(6):875-899.

Westover, A. N., and L. B. Marangell. 2002. A cross-national relationship between sugar consumption and major depression? *Depression and Anxiety* 16(3):118-120.

Wood, R. 1999. *The New Whole Foods Encyclopedia*. New York: Penguin.

Wynd, C. A. 2005. Guided health imagery for smoking cessation and long-term abstinence. *Journal of Nursing Scholarship* 37(3):245-250.

Yang, Q. 2010. Gain weight by "going diet"? Artificial sweeteners and the neurobiology of sugar cravings: Neuroscience 2010. *Yale Journal of Biology and Medicine* 83(2):101-108.

Yang, Y. J., S. J. Nam, G. Kong, and M. K. Kim. 2010. A case-control study on seaweed consumption and the risk of breast cancer. *British Journal of Nutrition* 103(9):1345-1353.

Zang, D. X. 1991. A self body double-blind clinical study of L-tryptophan and placebo in treated neurosis [article in Chinese]. [*Chinese Journal of Neurology and Psychiatry*] 24(2):77-80, 123-124.

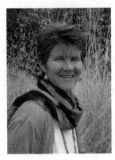

Trudy Scott, CN, has a nutrition practice that focuses on food, mood, and women's health. She lectures extensively, both at live events and via teleseminars. She is president of the National Association of Nutrition Professionals and a member of Anxiety Disorders Association of America, the Alliance for Addiction Solutions, and the National Alliance on Mental Illness. She lives in the greater Sacramento, CA, area.

Foreword writer **James Lake, MD**, is president of the International Network of Integrative Mental Health and author of the *Textbook of Integrative Mental Health Care*. He lives in Carmel, CA.

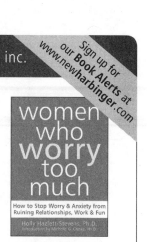
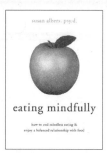
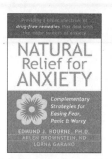
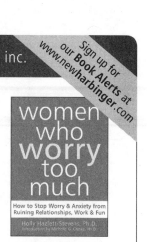
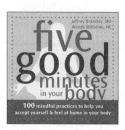
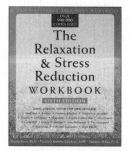
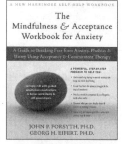

Index

A

about this book, 6–7

acupuncture, 163

addictions: alcohol, 64–65; benzodiazepine, 158; gluten, 73; sugar or carb, 57, 110–111

adrenal glands: blood sugar swings and, 41; caffeine consumption and, 61; dysfunction from overworked, 152–153; food sensitivities and, 71

agave nectar, 46, 48

agoraphobia, 24–25

alcohol consumption, 63–65; how to quit, 64–65; low blood sugar and, 64; nutritional deficiencies from, 63–64

allergies: brain or cerebral, 67; true or immediate food, 72. *See also* food sensitivities

aloe vera products, 107

American Heart Association, 49

American Journal of Psychiatry, 9

amino acids, 109–126; DPA or DLPA, 86, 119, 120; 5-HTP, 86, 113–114, 115–116, 125; food cravings and, 86–88, 110–111, 122–123; GABA, 86, 110, 111–113; glutamine, 55-56; guidelines for supplementing with, 123–124; precautions about using, 124–125; SSRI or MAOI medications and, 125–126; testing for levels of, 121–122; timeline for improvement

using, 126; tryptophan, 86, 114, 115–116, 125; tyrosine, 62, 86, 117, 118

animal protein, 17–21; fish and other seafood, 20–21; guidelines for eating, 21; organ meats, 33–34; poultry and eggs, 19; red meat, 18–19

antianxiety food solution diets, 10–14; bonus foods in, 33–35, 38–39; chart summarizing, 11–12; foods to avoid in, 31–33, 39; foods to include in, 14–31, 38; quantities/combinations of foods in, 35–36; recipe and food resources for, 36–37, 176; reference lists summarizing, 38–39

antidepressant medications, 125–126, 157

antifungal agents, 106

antigliadin antibodies, 77, 78

anxiety: caffeine and, 59–60; causes of, 5; conventional treatments for, x; digestive problems and, 90–91, 98–99; disorders related to, 4; gluten sensitivity and, 70–71, 74; individual nutrients for, 148–152; nicotine and, 65; research on diet and, 8–9; sleep problems and, 160; sugar consumption and, 43

Anxiety: Orthomolecular Diagnosis and Treatment (Prousky), 52

anxiety disorders: prevalence of, 3; types of, 4

miso, 35
molasses, 45
Monterey Bay Aquarium website, 21, 172
Mood Cure, The (Ross), 3, 5, 13, 110, 121, 124, 126
mood problems: gluten sensitivity and, 70–71, 74; histamine imbalances and, 88
multivitamin/multimineral supplements, 145–146
Murray, Michael, 52, 94

N

Naparstek, Belleruth, 163
natural approaches, 5–6
Natural Healing for Schizophrenia and Other Common Mental Disorders (Edelman), 131
Natural Relief for Anxiety (Bourne, Brownstein, and Garano), 161, 163
neurotransmitters, 57, 109–121; catecholamines, 117–118; cravings related to, 123; endorphins, 118–120; GABA, 111–113; serotonin, 113–117; testing levels of, 122. *See also* brain chemistry
New Whole Foods Encyclopedia, The (Wood), 36, 98
nicotine use, 65–66
Nielsen, Robin, 98
nonstarchy vegetables, 22–23
Nourishing Traditions (Fallon), 14, 37
nutrient deficiencies: alcohol consumption and, 63–64; anxiety related to, 6; medications causing, 157–158; refined sugar and, 43
nutrient excesses, 124
Nutrition and Mental Illness (Pfeiffer), 51, 52, 70, 127, 131
nuts, 25, 26, 84

O

obsessive-compulsive disorder (OCD), 4, 162
oligoantigenic diet, 83
olive oil, 24, 25, 105, 107
omega-3 fatty acids, 18, 118, 135–136, 142, 151
omega-6 fatty acids, 18, 136, 142, 151

onions, 105
OptiZinc, 138, 139
organ meats, 33–34
organic acids, 135
organic produce, 22–23
Osmond, Humphrey, 131
outdoor exercise, 159

P

P5P supplements, 140, 141
packaged foods. *See* processed foods
Paleo Diet, The (Cordain), 13
pancreatic enzyme deficiency, 100, 101
panic disorder, 4, 60
parasites, 103
Pemmican, 26
peripheral neuropathy, 140
pesticides, 22–23
Pfeiffer, Carl, 51, 52, 70, 127, 131, 157
Pfeiffer's law, 157
PharmaGABA, 112
phobias, specific, 4
Phytogenic Hormone Solution, The (McKenna), 152
Pizzorno, Joseph, 24, 52, 94
platelet testing of serotonin and the catecholamines, 122
PMS symptoms, 61
post-traumatic stress disorder (PTSD), 4
poultry, 19
prebiotics, 106
probiotics, 91, 105
processed foods: avoiding in antianxiety diet, 32, 81; sugars/sweeteners added to, 47–48
progesterone levels, 155
protein: amino acids in, 110; animal, 17–21; digestion of, 95; importance of, 17, 53, 110
Prousky, Jonathan, 52
pumpkin seeds, 25–26, 114, 139
pyroluria, 127–143; author's story, 2; biochemical description of, 127–128; conditions co-occurring with, 132–133; fatty acids for, 142; nutrients for treating, 138–142; prevalence and age of onset, 132; questionnaire about, 128–131; stress and, 143; symptoms of, 127, 128–131; testing for, 133–136; timeline for improving